"Dr. Sophia Apple is one of the most respected breast pathologists in the field. She has overcome the disability left from her childhood polio, gender, and the racial bias during her professional journey and came out the other side a strong, courageous, determined advocate for women and for those touched by breast cancer.

In her book, she takes the readers behind the scenes into the world of pathology, the science and practice of assigning a definitive diagnosis.

She shows us that pathologists are not faceless, but in fact, priceless in taking care of breast cancer patients.

Anyone diagnosed with breast cancer will appreciate Doctor Apple's clear explanations. Her knowledge is your power in battling with breast cancer."

— *Helena R. Chang, MD, PhD*
Surgical Oncologist and former Director of the Breast Cancer Program, *Revlon/UCLA Breast Center, and currently professor emerita at the David Geffen School of Medicine at UCLA.*

…as a medical professional who had seen cancer cell slides before, seeing my own confirmed my worst fears that indeed I had cancer. Seeing the wildly non-conforming cells, confirmed for me "that this was no joke, and it was GAME ON to fight this disease."

— *Anonymous Physician Assistant (PA), and breast cancer survivor*

ISBN: 9798837876981

Cover design by Hal and Sophia Apple
Production artwork for cover by Stephanie Robinson
For inquiries contact unseendoctor@gmail.com, or visit
DoctorSophiaOnline.com

Introduction

I thought about writing this book for 25 years but hesitated for several reasons. First, who will care to read this book since pathologists are unknown and unseen doctors? Out of sight, out of mind principle. Who will know the significance of this book since pathologists are not visible professionals in the medical field? Second, if this book is not visible, then who is going to buy the book? The practicality of a benefit versus risk factor hinders me to jump into writing such a book. It would take much time and effort to write a book that is not visible to the public.

My online searches find no such book. Books about pathology are often associated with forensic pathology, but this is a subspecialty of pathologists who mainly perform autopsies. Unfortunately, the field of speech pathology clouds over the medical practice of pathology, which makes our field even more ambiguous and hard to find through online searches.

Throughout my entire career as a breast pathology expert, only a rare number of patients want to know who their pathologist is in the context of their health care system. Unfortunately, patients often become aware of their pathologist only after receiving a "wrong diagnosis," and hence, begin to inquire about pathologists from a negative perspective, who they are, and what they do in the field of medicine.

Despite all the logic why I should not bother to write this book as I state above, this book needs to be written for several reasons. This book is written to record the profession of pathology, who we are, what we do, why we must exist in medicine, where we exist in the hospital setting, how we conduct our daily business, and when pathologists are necessary. I also write this book to thank all my thousands of patients whom I had a privilege to *"read"* (review and diagnose) their tissue samples and understand the pathology of each patient's individual breast disease, while enriching the experience of my medical practice. In breast pathology alone, there are hundreds, if not thousands of different diseases. Someone must write about our profession which has existed for over 120 years. No pain, no gain is a basis of my reasoning to finally write this book.

Finally, I write this book to overcome the fear of unknown and fear of failure. All the what-ifs, when said and questioned, are fears paralyzing us from doing the very things in life we seek. Fear has no warning, no boundaries, and no limits. It infiltrates quietly into the minds and destroys all dreams, hopes, and paralyzes all the potentials. What is the basis of fear? Is it the rejection or failure? Rejection by whom? What defines failure? What is success? What and who defines them? To whom the success is success and failure a failure? Fear is indeed meaningless and powerless. And to this reason, I decide to author this book.

Contents

I. What is pathology?

Chapter 1: History of the Pathology Profession

Drs. Van den Tweel and C. Taylor wrote an article in *Virchows Arch. 2010 Jul; 457(1): 3–10.*, a brief history of the pathology profession which summarizes how this discipline came about. Pathology literally means "to understand and study of the disease." In Latin, *ology* means study of, and *path* means disease. As expected, autopsies began the profession of pathology by examining the gross anatomy. In the mid-nineteenth century, the development of the microscope opened the new world of pathology by our founding father Virchow (1821–1902). During the 1850s, microscopic examination of tissue became prevalent, and the diagnostic application of processed tissue placed on glass slides became known as histopathology and changed our concept of diseases at a cellular level.

Understanding the etiology of disease is the foremost compelling cause in the field of pathology. This has been done in postmortem examinations as well as microscopic examinations specifically devoted to the correlation of disease in surgical specimens with clinical illness. By the late 1800s a great body of literature had accumulated on the gross anatomic diseases, and in the mid-1950s many of the diseases were characterized microscopically. Within a century and a half, dedicated pathologists continually discovered and documented the entire spectrum of the human diseases and developed new technology to study diseases further, including electron microscopy, immunofluorescence, special stains, immunohistochemical stains, in-situ hybridization, and now molecular pathology, which opens the world of nanometers.

Pathology is one of the oldest medical professions and for approximately 120 years has often co-existed with the history of surgery. Even today, surgeons and pathologists work together; surgeons cutting the diseased organs with the question, "What is wrong with this?" and pathologists answering specifically, "what it is and how it happened." The surgeon and pathologist are natural partners, moving in synchronized fashion as if we are dance partners. The surgeon receives the most attention, glory, and honor from the patient and the public. But it is the pathologist who often leads the surgeon where to go and where to cut, since the disease tissue vs. normal tissue is sometimes not distinctive. The greatest compliment as a pathologist I could receive from a surgeon was the statement, "You are my compass, a GPS guiding where I should go. Without you, I am lost."

Sir William Osler once mentioned, "As is our pathology, so is our practice; what the pathologists think today, the physician does tomorrow."

Pathologists are the "doctor's doctor." The job consists of great responsibility, naming the disease. Simply assigning a name to a disease is incredibly meaningful to the patient. This final diagnosis containing the name of the disease provides the next step, critical to research, treatment plans, and what to expect for survival and prognosis. Names have a profound influence on how we understand. Beyond a superficial designation of "What's in a name?" it gives the power to understand biases, supports decisions, diminishes subjectivity, and assuages uncertainty. In my opinion, pathology is the only field of medicine that offers the mastery of all specialties. Though pathologists do not see the patient or perform physical exams, the pathologist is the one who provides an ultimate name of the disease for the patient. Even with an autopsy, a pathologist is the last physician the deceased patient will encounter and will provide the final events that led to their demise. There is a classic joke among surgeons and pathologists: "Surgeons do not know anything but do everything and pathologists know everything but do nothing."

The field of medicine is like a body in concert. Some say, "Surgeons are the hands that remove the diseased part of an organ, internal medicine doctors figure out whether to ignore or further investigate the patient's complaints, and the pathologists are the brains behind the scenes." Pathologists do not see the patients and they are behind the scenes from the patient's point of view, and they are not known. Surgeons often imply that the "laboratory" will examine the tissue that was removed from the patient. It is then natural for some to picture a large space and septically clean machines that churn the tissue somehow and miraculously generate the name of the disease. Then, the surgeons and other doctors will do something to help the patients—such as prescribing pills, doing further surgery, or concocting chemotherapy regimens.

With a microscope, I can see indescribable beauty in the microscopic world not seen by a naked eye. This opened my eyes to the field of pathology in my second year of medical school as I experienced histology (study of normal tissue microscopically) and led me to decide that I should be a pathologist. The microscopy with light illuminating the beauty of the cells, variety in colors and structures, uniqueness of each organ at a cellular level fascinated me to know and learn more.

With the technology of a telescope, we can see a glimpse of uncountable and immeasurable stars in the sky. How many stars are in the universe? Astronomers estimate there are about 100 thousand million stars in the Milky Way alone, not counting the millions upon millions of other galaxies. Just as the countless stars in the sky and the discovery of new stars every day, we, the pathologists learn new things in the microscopic world every day. I look at different cells in the microscope and wonder how spectacular our body is made. In my personal opinion, the intricacy and complexity of how our body is made and functions is beyond my capability to fathom that it somehow is made accidentally.

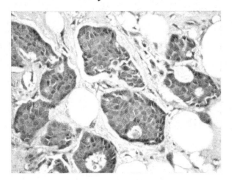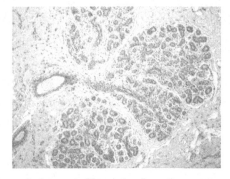

Left: Hematoxylin & Eosin-stained microscopic image of invasive breast cancer cells, infiltrating into normal fat and fibrous tissue. Compared to normal breast tissue, (right) showing organized lobules and ducts, the cancer cells are much larger, expanding the ducts by replicating uncontrollably by destroying normal structures.

Chapter 2:
What personalities does the field of pathology attract?

Most medical students do not become a doctor to become a pathologist. They do not even know the field of pathology. Most medical students want to become a doctor to see the patients who are in a desperate situation of need in their sickness, and then tangibly help them. In fact, most medical students have in their vision to become a doctor and a family practitioner, pediatrician, or surgeon who sees, touches, and listens to the patients and helps them by directly figuring out and alleviating their health problems. The "ideal doctor" is one who can help a patient with direct contact, treating a sick patient with compassion and good bedside manners.

Pathology is not a well-known specialty among medical students, partly because pathologists do not promote themselves well. Medical students often encounter a required course with a title of PATHOLOGY, in their second of year. Here, a student gets a glimpse of the profession with lectures consisting of inflammation of the body, micro-organisms causing diseases and neoplasms causing many diverse kinds of cancers. Pathology is the study of the essential nature of diseases, and the structural and functional changes and illnesses they cause. We learn what is wrong, and why it occurs. Medical students typically begin to realize that there are pathologists in their medical school when they see these medical doctors give presentations during basic lectures. Currently, medical students often learn basic medicine based on an "organ system" or "case based system," and not through didactic lectures in pathology courses. This will hinder exposure to pathology even further.

But this is how I first encountered the field of pathology during my second year of medical school. I also had a mindset of being a doctor who meets the patients and helps them out with my learned medical skills and knowledge.

For me, an intelligent pathologist introduced this field of pathology as he gave lectures. I am not the type to attend lectures because I learn not by auditory methods but visual methods. Especially in the early morning, I despise going to lectures. For one, I am not a morning person.

I must see and read the books in my own time in a completely quiet environment to learn and retain the information. My course in pathology began early in the morning at 8:00 am. He possessed a calming voice, and vast medical knowledge like a walking encyclopedia. He spoke an entirely different language—all in pathology words, explaining medicine at the cellular levels. I realized such an attractive field of medicine existed. I knew that I wanted to do the exact same thing as he was doing for my profession. I learned that the field of pathology is the essence and the core of medicine. This is the field that ties the disease and the etiology of a particular illness. It also ties basic science research and the practice of medicine. It requires my strongest talents which are visual acuity and memory. I can see things in the microscope—and identify what is the culprit of a specific disease. The new world opened for me—a visual world. It is immensely colorful, with numerous patterns, surprisingly beautiful and so challenging. There are countless diseases, so many new things to learn and so exciting to walk into the world of the microscope every day.

During my third and fourth years in medical school, I immediately encountered waves of patients who came to see their doctors. When asking why they came to the clinic or hospital, or even after arriving to the emergency department and acutely sick, commonly patients do not know, or cannot articulate why they came. A typical conversation can run like this:

Me: What brought you here today?
Patient: I am sick.
Me: Where is your pain?
Patient: All over.
Me: How long have you had the pain?
Patient: A long time.
Me: From a scale one to ten, one being little pain and ten being excruciating pain, how do you rate your pain today?
Patient: I don't know, maybe ten.
Me: Ten means you cannot even talk because you are in excruciating pain. Can you point to me exactly where is this pain?
Patient: I don't know. You are the doctor. You are supposed to figure it out and tell me what is wrong with me.

A vague complaint like this frustrates me very much. Equally frustrating is doctors will ultimately deal with social issues such as where to place the patients who do not have a home or a place to go after they are discharged from the hospital; or complex family and social issues dealing with elderly; or child abuse situations.

During my training, I felt most of the internal medicine doctors were using their time to deal with these kinds of situations rather than using their medical skills. I applaud internal medicine or family doctors who deal with chronic illness such as alcoholism, diabetes, high blood pressures, and chronic pains, day in and day out. While the pathologist gladly allows primary care doctors to face the actual patients, it is the pathologist who provides liver enzyme analysis for the alcoholic patients and monitors A1c level for diabetic patients, behind a curtain. Without a pathologist running the clinical laboratory, primary care doctors cannot well serve the patients. And therefore, chronic disease management is often driven by the laboratory medicine overseen by pathologists.

Even though pathologists do not see patients on a day-to-day basis, a pathologist considers what the best care for a particular patient might be, working alone in a quiet environment.

The surgeon cuts the diseased organs, and the interventional radiologist performs the core needle or fine needle aspiration biopsy samples. The tissue is brought to the pathologist after others handle all the required face-to-face time with the patient. It is the pathologist who sits down in front of the microscope, looks at what other doctors have procured and will know the cause and the mystery of the disease of a patient before anyone else.

The elaborate structural difference in each cell is so intriguing to me that I do not know why other people do not get excited when they see the microscopic world. I also love the fact that I can have a coffee whenever I want one and go to the bathroom anytime I need to go, unlike the surgeon who must remain in their operation room because the patient is under the anesthesia, and they must use the operation time judiciously, sacrificing their own physical needs. The surgeon does not have freedom to go and use the bathroom anytime there is the need and drink coffee when they feel like having one. These are the luxuries a pathologist might enjoy during the days in their quiet offices.

The microscope is the main instrument for anatomic pathologists. It is their instrument to use day in and day out. Oddly, microscopes are frequently staged to be seen in the background in hospital settings for news and entertainment stories, but a microscope is the pathologist's instrument. Microscope connotates intelligence, perhaps. Recently, digital pathology has begun replacing certain usage of the microscope with computer monitors by scanning the slides for use in digital technology. But I still see the visual images which I love.

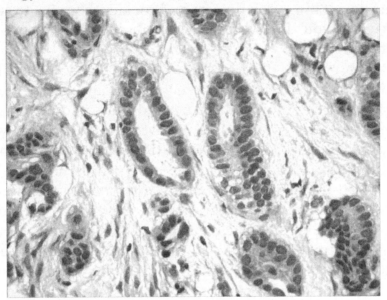

Hematoxylin & Eosin-stained breast cancer cells forming round structures with central holes; gland formation. This is an example of a well-differentiated invasive ductal carcinoma.

Most pathologists are introverts like me. Recently I read an incredible book, *Quiet*, by Susan Cain. This book illuminates how much our insightful, quiet, and effective introverts are needed among our culture of extraverts who cannot stop talking. In her book, she writes, "Talkative people, for example, are rated smarter, better looking, more interesting, and more desirable as friends. Velocity of speech counts as well as volume: we rank fast talkers as more competent and likable than slow ones. The same dynamics apply in groups, where research shows that the voluble are considered smarter than the reticent—even though there's zero correlation between the gist and gab and good ideas."

There are obviously fast speakers and extroverts among pathologists, but the vast majority of pathologists are introverts who recharge their batteries when they are alone, not socializing or talking to others. We enjoy working deliberately, focusing on the power of concentration without the lures of popularity, recognition, and fame from their patients.

Majority of pathologists are quiet, smart, nerdy, and meticulous with obsessive-compulsive personality traits because our profession attracts such people. The downside is we pathologists become overlooked, and not recognized. Multiple surgery colleagues have told me, "It is too bad that patients do not bring you flowers and cookies they give to surgeons like me, because you deserve these. You rescue the patient's life by giving the correct diagnosis."

Yes, it is true patients do not recognize me because I am a faceless doctor behind the scenes, but I will take that any day over the burden of disturbing my concentration of thinking, and peace in quietness.

It is comforting such a person like Mahatma Gandhi is known as an introvert and shy. According to his autobiography we learn of his creative and effective leadership. In his own words he said, "I have naturally formed the habit of restraining my thoughts. A thoughtless word hardly ever escaped my tongue or pen. Experience has taught me that silence is part of the spiritual discipline of a votary of truth. We find so many people impatient to talk. All this talking can hardly be said to be any benefit to the world. It is so much waste of time. My shyness has been in reality my shield of buckler. It has allowed me to grow. It has helped me in my discernment of truth."

Chapter 3:
Why did I become a pathologist?

Originally, I wanted to practice Rehabilitation and Physical Medicine. This motivated me to become a doctor from the beginning because I have polio in my right leg since age two. Polio is caused by poliovirus resulting in mobility paralysis and atrophy of muscles of the affected limb. I particularly wanted to focus my work on children with mobility disabilities since I can connect with them the most. Every time I encountered a person with mobility disabilities, my heart would sink to the point I could not even talk and teared up. I know the depth of pain that person goes through every day, both physically and emotionally. Even to this day, I cannot accustom myself to deal with the difficulties in my own physical limitations or deal with emotional pains that accompany the disability. I will rather avoid seeing them and escape the suffocating pain I also feel every day of my life. Gradually, I came to realize the blind cannot help other blind. A hungry person cannot help hunger. I sensed that I need to leave the field of rehabilitation medicine to those who can help these patients, and not to feel their pains of being disabled to the point of paralysis in depression.

I come from a humble childhood, born in Korea, the second daughter of three children from educated parents. The first child was a daughter, and my parents wanted a boy. My mother certainly thought I was a boy since I moved so much in her womb. A long-awaited boy had to wait a bit longer since I was another girl. Growing up, I had little attention from my family since I was just another girl and a middle child. The only time I received praise for my existence was because "my brother was subsequently born after me," as if I had a power to determine which sex would follow me. Because no one paid much attention to me, I was free to think whatever I wanted to think and do. I was a strong child, independent and free. When I was two years old (Korea counts nine months in a womb one year, so a 2-year-old in Korea is one year old in America), I was already able to walk and run but hot water accidentally spilled onto my legs. After my recovery from the burns, I was found to have polio affecting mainly my right leg, and some in the left leg. Luckily, I can walk with a long leg brace on the right leg, with a shoe lift. The polio affects motor function without sensory loss, causing atrophy of the muscle and unequal growth of the leg length. Due to the shorter length of the right leg, the spine curvature is exaggerated, and hypertrophy of the left side occurred. Most Asians not born in the US who had a disability would have little or no opportunity to become a functional person in the society, especially back then. Going to school was difficult, let alone becoming a physician. Thanks to my parents who never gave up immigrating to the US for me to even hope for an educational opportunity. I came to the States when I was 13 years old and enrolled in a junior high public school in New York City, a tough environment. I did not speak English at all. It was truly a humble start, but I never gave up the opportunity to be educated. Education for me was the only ticket which might free me from this miserable and expected consequence of disability, and I might at least lessen the burden from my family to support me.

I wanted to become a doctor ever since I was five years old. I remember dissecting a large frog my brother caught one day just to see what is inside the frog. I was fascinated by the movement of the heart and all the intricate, wet internal organs.

It was difficult to learn English and it took almost three years for me to understand and talk. I am still conscious of speaking and writing English with correct grammar and sentence structures. But I think English is my most comfortable language since living in the States for 47 years. I can speak some Korean and Japanese (I grew up in Japan for over three years) and mostly English, but none perfectly.

Medical school was difficult, not in terms of understanding and mastering the concepts but in terms of physical challenges and limitations during the third and fourth years in clinical rotations. The memory is palpable: *I tag along with "attending" physicians in hospitals as they personally check on the status of their patients, called ROUNDS. Rounding early each morning before sunrise, long hours retracting (holding open with both my arms) the incision sites in the surgery operation room, urgent and speedy movements needed in the emergency department, constant changes, and fear of unknowns in rotational schedules require me to experience the different physical demands in the fields of clinical medicine. I can never walk fast to keep up with the attendings and residents and often miss their key points and plans to treat the patients because I am always behind them and desperate to stay within eyesight of the group with white coats. On top of this, most doctors are males who discuss their plans for surgeries while they change in and out of scrubs in the men's locker rooms. When I join them in the operating room (OR), I feel left out on what they have already discussed, naturally fall behind, and I feel inadequate which they attribute to me being a woman.*

So, it was not just the disability but being a woman made my career in medicine doubly hard. I refused to listen or to hear these nonsenses but pushed on through the mountains of challenges and barriers, no matter how difficult it was because I had to. To compensate I studied doubly hard, making sure to know my anatomy and any esoteric pimping questions the attending physicians might ask me. Failure was not an option to me. And my God gave me the strength, power, and wisdom every day of my life.

The field of pathology is attractive to me, mostly because of the intellectual element, and I enjoy doing the job immensely. The most enjoyable hobby becoming an actual job: a perfect marriage. I can sit down and look through the microscope which takes me to a different world that I never knew existed. The intricate patterns, the colors and the beauty of cells are phenomenal. It is the world in the midst of quietness, ability to think deeply into the core of medicine without the fuss or distractions, freedom of work schedules without getting tied to the rigid OR schedules or patients waiting in the clinic, ability to detach emotional aspects of patients' sadness due to their illness because I usually cry when the patient talks about their pains, and to have a better work-life balance than most other fields in medicine. Yes, a pathologist gets calls at nights and on weekends, but those times are much fewer in number than other physicians. Ironically, the pathologists see the greatest number of patients daily than any other physicians. No other doctor can see hundreds of patients per day, simply due to the physical and time limitations but as a pathologist, we can look at hundreds of patient samples a day, easily. When feeling like I made a great diagnosis and my brain takes off and rises into the clouds of a pride trip, I look back where I came from which makes me humble and thankful that I get to be here, practicing pathology, patients allowing me to look at their tissues, and participating in the most important aspect of medicine: naming the diseases, a first step into the road of recovery.

Chapter 4:
Areas of specialty within pathology

Most people approach others by saying "hello" or "hi," and the very next question is, "What do you do?" I consider how to respond countless times in life, and depending on the circumstances or who asks, I carefully respond accordingly. When saying, "I am a pathologist," I often get another question. "What do pathologists do, exactly?" Those who ask this question are often inquisitive and care to find out what I do for a living. Others often assume a pathologist does autopsies and forensic medicine, thanks to the media and television shows glorifying pathologists who figure out the crime scenes and investigate deaths; "know-it-all" types mostly related to forensics. The classic television show about the pathologist is *Quincy* from the late 70s. More recently, there are other shows, one featuring a gorgeous woman as a pathologist playing a tough role sorting out the events and causes of deaths. There are hundreds of novels about pathologists who solve the etiology and sequences of death. Although autopsy is a part of the job for certain pathologists, it is a small portion of the total work most pathologists perform. I rarely perform autopsy in my practice and autopsy is the least favorable part of my job.

There are multiple specialties in pathology, divided mainly into two subdivisions: anatomic pathology (AP) and clinical pathology (CP).

Anatomic pathology (AP) is composed of different disciplines; autopsy, surgical pathology, cytopathology, neuropathology, and dermatopathology. Forensic pathologists are the medical examiners in the county coroner's office who do the autopsy to determine the cause of death and provide a death certificate. They are the final medical doctor a patient sees. This doctor determines the most objective causes of death.

Surgical pathology deals with tissue diagnosis of all body systems. Cytopathology is fluid diagnosis dealing with the cellular level. Neuropathology is study of the brain. Dermatopathology is study of skin disease. (The details of surgical and cytopathology will be discussed later in the book). Within surgical pathology, there are pathology subspecialties (usually in academic settings). These pathologists sign out (render a diagnosis) with expertise in each organ system: breast, head and neck, thorax and lung, soft tissue and bone, endocrine, obstetrics and gynecology, genitourinary, and gastrointestinal with pancreas and liver. In community hospitals, the pathologist often looks at all organ systems and practices general pathology.

Clinical pathology (CP) is composed of laboratory medicine. There are mainly four parts in laboratory medicine which are chemistry, blood bank, microbiology and hematopathology. Within CP, there are also cytogenetic laboratories performing multitudes of tests, including Chromosome analysis for prenatal samples, peripheral blood, bone marrow, lymphomas and solid tumors, Fluorescence In Situ Hybridization (FISH) assays and microarray assays for congenital (pre- and postnatal) disorders tests; all commonly performed in these labs.
Molecular pathology is now becoming more visible, and this subspecialty deals with genomics, and more recently, "precision medicine." At different institutions, molecular pathology is under either anatomic or clinical pathology. It is now becoming large enough as its own entity at certain institutions, sometimes becoming its own subdivision of pathology.

As one can see, under the umbrella of pathology many subspecialties and subdivisions work together to deliver the most current, comprehensive, and useful information and diagnostic tests to serve the patient populations. In most hospital settings the pathology department is one of the largest in terms of staff numbers, aside from nursing. Numerous career opportunities within the pathology department includes laboratory technicians, cytotechnicians, histotechnicians, physician assistants (PA), and other licensed laboratory personnel, aside from pathologists.
To become a pathologist, one must finish medical school and complete a residency program. The choices are to be an anatomic or a clinical pathologist, each requiring two years of training. A majority combine anatomic and clinical pathology, taking four years of training. To practice as a pathologist, one needs to obtain a medical practice license from their state, and a pathology license(s) by passing the pathology board examination(s). Most pathologists have both anatomic

and clinical pathology licenses, especially in community practice settings that normally require both parts for daily pathology practice.

The subspecialties beyond anatomic and clinical pathology require a "fellowship" of one to two additional years of specialized training and a separate license. These additional fellowship trainings and licenses include cytopathology, hematopathology, dermatopathology, molecular genetic pathology, transfusion medicine, neuropathology, forensic pathology, and pediatric pathology. More recently, a new "clinical informatics" fellowship program has opened in various academic institutions.

There are differences in salaries in all subspecialties in pathology; namely, the highest salary is often among dermatopathology, and hence competition for theses fellowships is more competitive.

In 2017, it is reported that the number of active pathologists in the US is 12,839. (1.43% of all US physicians). According to a *JAMA* article in 2019 written by G. Lundberg (*JAMA Netw Open. 2019;2(5)*), only about 3% of graduating American medical students entered pathology and decreasing in a total number from 2007 by 17%.

There are mainly two types of career paths for pathologists: academic and community practice. More recently, large commercial labs are opening and growing in number, such as LabCorp and Quest Diagnostics. All these have both anatomic and clinical pathology practices.

I practiced in a major university hospital and became known as an academic pathologist. Now, I am a practicing pathologist in a large community hospital as a part-timer. Community pathology practices are typically in a smaller hospital, have minimal or no affiliations with university hospitals, and little to no teaching or training of pathology residents and medical students. There are more community pathologists in the US than academic pathologists. The differences between the academic and community (private) practices according to what the *Student Doctor Network* published back in 2011 are as follows:

Academic Practice

You have residents who can gross specimens, do autopsies, and write the reports for you.

You have to teach the residents and medical students.

Give lectures (make PowerPoints) and microscope teaching sessions (e.g., unknown cases).

Research and publishing. In some academic institutions, every attending has to show certain number of papers or academic work every 1–2 years for promotion.

Will be assigned academic rank which is promoted based on certain criteria (assistant, associate, and then full professor).

Less payment in salary (120–250K).

Have the opportunity to subspecialize and sign out cases belonging to your area of interest only.

Good for people who live to work (if you want pathology to take your whole life, spending time at home working on publications and teaching lectures).

Because of the competition in research, publication and others, the environment is not very friendly.

Private Practice

No residents. You do things on your own with some sort of help from pathology assistants.

No teaching. Just focus on your sign out.

Make diagnosis and write your report. No home preparation for lectures.

No research or publication.

Enjoy the weekends and enjoy life!

No academic ranking.

> You are (staff pathologist) forever. In the middle of your career however, you can apply to become a lab director. That's it!
>
> More payment (usually exceeds 200–300K+). The payment can be higher than that when you become a lab director.
>
> Less chance to sign out cases of your own interest only, but still can develop interest or expertise in one area. Also, you may be required to do CP work besides just AP.
>
> Good for people who work to live (sign out and go home; nothing more to worry about).
>
> Usually more friendly and "benign" environment as there is less competition among the staff.
>
> *Student Doctor Network, 2011*

I cannot add or disagree too much from the lists above. Both academic and community practices involve doing surgical pathology most of the time in anatomic pathology. Surgical pathology consists of doing frozen sections, cutting gross specimens and analyzing surgical permanent specimens, providing the preliminary and final diagnosis.

In addition to full time pathology positions in hospital settings or a commercial laboratory, pathologists may also choose to work as a per-diem or in a part-time role. Other positions for pathologists exist in major scientific corporations or drug companies such as Amgen, in positions such as researchers, medical directors, or medical consultants, without practicing medicine. Pathologists can also teach medical courses at medical, dental, and nursing schools, or teach at the college or high school level.

Chapter 5:
What does a pathologist do in a typical day?

Patients and surgeons are often anxious to receive the diagnosis from the pathologist and surgeons routinely ask in jest, "Why does it take so long to get the result?" and the pathologist may want to reply, "You wanted the result yesterday, a day before the surgery happened." Surgeons commonly wonder why their pathologist takes so much time to generate a pathology report containing the final diagnosis. This is quite understandable because their patient is behind them, waiting. Waiting is the hardest discipline to be perfected by most of us but required for pathologists to do their job correctly.

"Patients are called patients because they need to be patient," one of my mentors said. Each day must seem like a month to the patient who anticipates answers from their doctor. I hate waiting, but this waiting is critical to each patient who needs to think about the next step in their life. Many patients consider a cancer diagnosis as terminal, and one needs to put things in order in case death is an imminent fact. Cancer diagnosis is perhaps the most reality-shaking news.

One of the most frustrating components of our job is the lack of understanding from many surgeons and other clinicians who still do not understand the complexity of a pathologist's job. We juggle and handle thousands of patients' samples, including cutting the tissue samples, participating in what appears to be countless hospital tumor boards, performing critically urgent frozen sections, politely answering phone calls from clinicians, rushing to operation rooms for first-hand knowledge of complex orientations of surgeons' cut specimens, craving our moments of uninterrupted quiet time to review our patients' slides, ordering necessary ancillary tests, researching and looking up the newest criteria and updated literature on difficult cases, carefully finessing and clarifying our comments and microscopic examination reports to be understood by the surgeons and clinicians so they will not be offended by a pathologist telling them what to do and how to manage the next step, answering questions and reviewing slides from other pathology colleagues, replying to urgent emails, attending required hospital meetings, and teaching residents and medical students who study under the pathologist working in an academic setting.

To surgeons and clinicians, the patient is their client. But to pathologists, the surgeons and clinicians are the client. It is our goal to satisfy the clients by providing the best service with speed and utmost accuracy. Most surgeons and clinicians think their job is much more important and stressful as they work on the front line, deal directly with their patients, and not appreciative to what the pathologist faces daily "behind the curtain." The pressure for the pathologist is undeniable. We cannot make any mistake, and indirectly we see countless more patients as we review immense numbers of patients' samples; more than clinical colleagues may ever know.

It is important for the pathologist to maintain the workflow in a natural order. Frozen sections always take priority, RUSH cases are read first thing in the mornings. This is followed by reviewing immunohistochemical stains which require an additional day from the previous cases to wrap up the final diagnosis, then addressing any known urgent cases from the clinical colleagues who need to be informed of certain cases, then finally we review the routine cases. I usually finish my day with the core biopsies, FNA, and then excisional biopsies.

Sometimes we get a request to expedite Very Important Person (VIP) cases. Ironically, VIP cases are blundered more easily. Inevitably, singling out a case from the routines causes more angst in handling, and interrupts the well-greased system. It takes a toll for everyone to selectively pick and choose the VIP case to be seen first. It is best to have all cases as routine, and not distinguish VIP cases. To me, all patients are VIP without exception. I deplore disrupting the usual order of the allocation of focus due to VIP requests. I imagine cutting in line at Heaven's door by a VIP, and is that even allowed? Everyone is created equally without exception, and everyone will get the equal focus and concentrated time for the pathologist to look at the cases.

Chapter 6:
Why do pathologists not see patients?

It has been a tradition that pathologists do not directly see the patient face to face. Pathologists are considered as a consultant to other physicians. We are sometimes known as "unseen doctors," the brain behind clinical doctors. A patient who comes seeking a medical doctor makes an appointment and tells the doctor their symptoms and discomforts. Medical doctors then formulate what might be the cause of the illness; this is called the clinical differential diagnosis. To "rule in" or "rule out" many possible differential diagnoses, many tests are needed such as imaging, including (Computed Tomography scan (CT), mammogram, Ultrasound (US), Magnetic Resonance Imaging (MRI); or blood tests from the clinical laboratory within the pathology department, and even obtaining tissue samples. Aside from imaging, each and every body fluid and tissue sample ends up in the domain of the pathology department. The pathologist provides a final diagnostic report to explain the cause of the illness in the patient. Naming the exact cause of an illness is the most critical component to manage further treatment for the patient. If the pathologist provides an incorrect diagnosis, every health care provider and treatment regimen at this point forward is likely on the wrong path. In medicine, we sometimes hear pathologists are the CIA, radiologists are the FBI, surgeons are the frontline infantry warriors, and oncologists are the commanders of chemical weaponry. If the CIA and FBI get the wrong intelligence, all other fields will go down the drain and head down the wrong pathway. Fortunately, pathologists are traditionally not the target of medical lawsuits, unlike other specialists such as surgeons, but the stakes are high—if a pathologist makes a mistake, the resulting payout for medical malpractice may be enormous and more importantly, tragic for the patient who receives incorrect and harmful medical treatment.

A particular and small subset of pathologists frequently see patients to perform a procedure called *Fine Needle Aspiration (FNA)*. An FNA is either by palpation or by ultrasound imaging. The needle size is tiny, usually 25 gauge and hence called fine needle. The benefit of using this tiny sized needle is to obtain cells of interest with minimal bleeding since blood obscures the cells, and yields "drying artifact." FNA procedure is useful for thyroid, breast and any superficial lumps and bumps that are easily accessible. These FNA procedures are done by cytopathologists, who require an additional license and fellowship training. I am one of these cytopathologists and have the privilege of meeting patients who required an FNA during my career. Amazing patients in my brief encounters taught me their view and philosophy in life.

One such patient lost almost half of her face due to head and neck cancer. She came to the FNA clinic because of a tumor regrowth in her scar site. She was severely disfigured and shocking to see. She wore a hat and wrapped half her face with a scarf. She lived in fear that people would look at her with disbelief and disgust. She was in pain and shame. The extent people prefer to stay living by paying such a costly price is astonishing. Life is indeed priceless. She hesitated to show the lump or allow me to procure samples. As she began unwrapping her face and revealing her scar, she was crying. It was difficult to disguise the horror in my body language. I held her hand. She knew that I had my own sets of physical limitations and knew I had gone through emotional and mental pain not too dissimilar to hers. (I have polio on my right leg). There was unspoken language of understanding and compassion with each other. We had a special bond at that moment and there was a mutual understanding of enormous burdens we each carried in our daily lives. This kind of human understanding needs no words and felt between people who go through certain amounts of pain. After the procedure, I hugged her without a word. This patient helped me realize why I must suffer from my own physical limitations.

A second patient is a man who had lost his wife after her long breast cancer battle a week prior to our encounter. He came with a skin nodule in his arm. While I was preparing to do an FNA, he gave me a beautiful smile and told me his story, saying how much he loved his wife. His wife was his best friend, confidant, and love of his life. He said he does not see his life without her and would like to join her in Heaven. He ultimately knew that this lump was the pathway to go to Heaven. He believed in his heart that without a doubt he had a "cancer," and he welcomed the idea wholeheartedly. Indeed, he had a chloroma which is a rare, malignant tumor made up of granulocyte precursor cells. It is also called granulocytic sarcoma or extramedullary myeloblastoma and is usually associated with myeloblastic leukemia. He was in peace with his own death, even looking forward to it, and meeting his lover in Heaven.

I realized love transcends the power of death and nothing is stronger than love.

There are certain patients who provided incredible life lessons in my career. I am most grateful to meet such wonderful human beings. Nothing in life such as wealth, power, social status, degrees, pleasures, loyalty, fame is more important than the human encounters such as these.

While the quiet bunch of pathologists enjoy our undisturbed thinking time contemplating, it is also good to realize face-to-face contact builds trust and is an important part of patient care, not only between pathologists and clinicians but also to our patients. Although it is not a traditional practice, I think it is good to introduce occasional face-to-face time with patients as a consultant to patients in the medical arena. Eventually, it is not good enough to just sit with a microscope and computer to generate the final pathology report. I welcome the eventual opportunity for patients to meet and choose their pathologists as they choose surgeons or other medical doctors of their choice. This can be a logical evolution in patient care as patients become more aware of the role of their pathologist. Occasionally, a patient may call me and in rare cases ask to meet me.

One breast cancer patient scheduled time with me and asked to see what her enemy looked like under the microscope. It was a powerful moment for her to meet and see her enemy which was in her imagination only. To her, it was a life changing experience to face her unknown destroyer called cancer cells and she exclaimed, "Now I can see, not just imagine these cells in my mental mind, and I have seen the face of my enemy to fight back!" She added, "Why is this not done as a part of the road to recovery for the cancer patient program, to visualize what the cancer actually looks like, to see the enemy face to face?" A picture can express a thousand words. *"I will meditate on the images I saw and have courage to fight, rather than fighting back at an abstract thing called cancer," she concluded.*

I am happy to be of help to her and welcome the idea of the pathologist contributing to the road of cancer recovery treatment. I also find that each contact with a patient that I experience brings such joy and different learning moments. People bring different perspectives, purposes and meanings in this life and memorable moments in my career. I will always remember each patient I met face to face more than a thousand "great diagnoses" I ever made.

Including pathologists to build team dynamics in breast cancer patient care, and to enhance better and safer ways of communication among different specialties such as multidisciplinary conferences, is important. Bringing surgeons, oncologists, radiologists, radiation oncologists, primary care physicians, psychiatric and mental health care workers, social workers, and pathologists together to focus on breast cancer, one patient at a time, is critical to deliver the best care for that individual. This activity of breast multidisciplinary conferences is already in place for many hospitals for breast cancer patients, providing comprehensive care. I remember how much I learned through each session and recognize how important it is to care for the patient's entire care; physical, emotional, and spiritual aspect of health care. Appropriate diet, sleep, family support, social support, transportation situation/limitation, are all important aspects of health care we physicians need to understand and sympathize better, not just discuss the diseases and cancers. We must also understand and embrace cultural sensitivity for each patient as a required element of health care. Certain patients want to know every aspect of their breast cancer to make informed decisions; other patients trust doctors entirely, and others are suspicious of physicians and speculate ideas and unusual preconceptions about doctors without a logical reason.

To those patients who want to know every aspect of their breast cancer or to those simply curious about what their cancers look like, the opportunity exists to make a faceless pathologist become history of the past. If a patient wants to see their pathologist and observe the slide under a microscope, such opportunity should be encouraged in the future. Let us consider structural changes within our health care system to accomplish this change, including scheduling of appointments, fees for this service, and discussion among forward-thinking pathologists, clinicians, and health care administrators.

II. Human tissue and "the lab"

Chapter 7:
What is a frozen section?

Surgeries often involve on-the-spot decisions to remove an organ such as a cancer or transplant, cease a surgery, expand the scope of a surgery, and more. This is when the surgeon needs the expertise of a pathologist, who oversees the frozen section and then determines the diagnosis. These frozen section situations are the most frequent purposes of night and weekend calls for a pathologist.

Frozen section is one of the responsibilities of surgical pathology under the umbrella of anatomic pathology. Another name for frozen section is cryosection, which is a technique used for rapid diagnosis intraoperatively (during the surgery) for critical patient management. The technique is done by quickly freezing the tissue provided by the surgeon from the operation table, cutting thin slices, and placing the thin layer of tissue onto a glass slide, then rapidly staining the slide tissue with Hematoxylin and Eosin (H&E) to visualize the tissue under the microscope. H&E stain is a standard stain all pathology laboratories use. It stains in blue/purple by Hematoxylin stain, and pink/red colors by Eosin stain. Ideally, the cutting, staining, and reading of the slide for the frozen section should take place within 20 minutes for a single specimen. If there are multiple frozen specimens, the 20-minute rule does not apply. The result of the frozen section is directly communicated to the operation room surgeon by the pathologist using intercom or telephone to deliver a verbal report expeditiously.

Frozen section inevitably introduces artifacts, and hence, the sections from the tissue are not ideal as the permanent section, which is placed in a formalin fixation, then onto paraffin-embedded tissue sections on glass slides. Therefore, it should be used only in specific situations where the surgeon may need to alter the management of the patient immediately.

Clinical indications of performing a frozen section includes identification of the tumor or tissue type, margin of the tumor, extent of the disease, and to determine further staging during surgery or not. For example, surgeon may send a piece of tissue from a large mass from the retroperitoneal area (behind the organ adjacent to the vertebral column) for frozen section, and the pathologist will tell the surgeon what it is. If it is a lymph node tissue, and suspicious for lymphoma, this needs to be communicated to the surgeon. Lymphoma workup task is done by the pathologist and the surgery in progress will normally stop. If the tissue is cancerous (sarcoma or carcinoma), the surgeon will cut out the mass with clean margins. Ultimately, a pathologist's examination of the tissue by rapid technique is critical for a surgeon to take the next step.

Frozen section should not be used if:
1. it has no immediate implications for decision making,
2. the mass is very small, and the tissue is needed for additional/ancillary permanent processing (requiring extensive study for diagnosis by sending it to a molecular lab),
3. the tissue is fatty or bony/heavily calcified since the cryostat (machine that will cut the frozen tissue) cannot cut the specimens, and,
4. the patient has a known infectious condition such as HIV, tuberculosis, or Creutzfeldt-Jakob disease (CJD), hepatitis B or C and COVID-19 because the entire staff working in the frozen section area and the cryostat itself will be contaminated. It takes minimal 4–6 hours to decontaminate the cryostat. Cryostat consists of a sharp knife to cut the frozen tissue. Since there is a danger of cutting the technician's or pathologist's hands/fingers with every use of a sharp instrument, it is necessary to decontaminate all machines including the cryostat after a known infectious specimen. During decontamination period, pathology work needs to cease, and contamination in a rare situation may require portions of the building to be shut down.
5. A frozen section should also not be used if it is for a diagnostic purpose for the first time. For the very initial diagnosis of breast cancer, the most common and accurate method is a core needle biopsy performed in the radiology department by the radiologist. Frozen section diagnosis has many limitations: lack of time to confirm the diagnosis by using immunohistochemical stains,

frozen section artifacts including difficulty cutting fatty tissue and tissue folding, and many breast diseases mimic invasive carcinoma. In many cases, the diagnosis should be done on permanent tissue specimens.

Most pathologists find the frozen section task the most challenging part of their work due to the urgent need of surgeons in the operation room to take next immediate steps while their patient lies on the operating table, and the high stakes in making any mistake. The pathologist must make a swift and correct decision, and it is based on the frozen section slide which is typically not as crisp and clear as the permanent section.

The permanent section is tissue routinely handled by grossing and tissue processing. The permanent sections do not show artifacts such as freezing, folding, bubbles and chattering artifacts commonly seen in the frozen sections, so permanent section is the most common, preferred, and ideal way to examine the tissue for diagnosis by a pathologist. The permanent sections also do not have limitations for fatty and bony tissues. Bony tissue includes a decalcification step to cut this hard tissue. We simply put a part of the bone into a decal solution overnight to make it soft enough to be able to cut by a knife.

College of American Pathologists (CAP) guidelines for frozen section turn-around-time (TAT) is within 20 minutes, 90% of the time, for a single block of a single specimen. TAT starts when the tissue is received by the pathology laboratory. It includes accessioning the patient's case, printing the label for the frozen section slide, examining the tissue sent for frozen, putting the tissue with the correct orientation into the cold freezing chuck and freezing the tissue with an embedding media called Tissue-Tek O.C.T Compound. It stands for Optimal Cutting Temperature, and the high viscosity results in fast freezing that is ideal for cutting the frozen tissue into 4–6 micron-thin sections, putting the tissue onto the slide, and manually staining the slide with H&E stains. This should all take place within 15 minutes. Only 5 minutes remain for the pathologist to "read" the case, make a diagnosis, and communicate back to the surgeon and the team who are waiting in the operation room. There is no time for error in all these steps.

Accuracy of the frozen section diagnosis is estimated to be 97.8%, which is high. Pathologists can defer to answer the frozen section diagnosis when the case is too difficult to diagnose. The deferral rate should be under 5%. Miscommunications can develop between the pathologists and the surgeons and occurs approximately 2.7% of the time. It is especially important to be concise, clear, and skillful when communicating the results of the frozen section because of the significant and immediate impact to the patient's care in the operation room.

One of the classic examples of miscommunication occurred as follows: The surgeon cut a piece of tissue from the neck lymph node and asks over the intercom, "What is it?" The pathologist did all the necessary preparation and examination, and verbally communicates over the intercom, "No metastatic carcinoma in the lymph node." The beginning "No" portion of the audio sentence is cut off over the intercom, so the surgeon hears, "Metastatic carcinoma in the lymph node."

This was a case of an "atypical follicular cells in the thyroid" from a patient's earlier fine needle aspiration (FNA) diagnosis, which means the patient may have 5–25% chance of having a thyroid cancer. In this case, the surgeon heard "metastatic carcinoma in the lymph node" from the pathologist, which means it is confirmed that the patient surely has a thyroid cancer. The surgeon proceeded to remove the entire thyroid glands and dissected the neck lymph nodes from the patient. After surgery, the permanent tissue sample showed no thyroid cancer and no metastatic carcinoma in all lymph nodes.

We all know that verbal communication has limits; it has been said body language is 90% of our communication and verbal language is 10% of the communication. Verbal communication by either phone or intercom is even more limiting and prone to technical difficulties. Face-to-face communication between a surgeon and pathologist is not practical and rarely done intraoperation. In this scenario, the operation room and the pathology anatomic laboratory are separate, and often quite remote with significant physical distance. The pathologist also must take valuable time to "scrub in" before entering an operation room. Skillful communication from the first scenario is to say, "NEGATIVE for metastatic carcinoma in the lymph node," and ask the surgeon to repeat back what they just heard. Surgeons seldom follow the direction from pathologists, in my opinion, but I have experienced a few surgeons who repeat back what I say without me asking, to protect the patient care and I always appreciate these surgeons.

It is also important for the pathologist to read out the patient's name and the medical record numbers (two different identifiers of the patient) before blurting out the frozen section diagnosis through intercom or phone because there are many operation rooms simultaneously asking for frozen sections and calling the pathologist at the same time. It is not unusual to receive multiple frozen section requests from five or even ten different operation rooms at the same time because operations in a hospital generally start at the same time, usually about 7:00 am and often finish at the same time. A pathology lab can become hectic when performing frozen sections within the 20-minute deadline while keeping track of which patient's frozen section result is communicated to which operation room. One can imagine the disaster if a "positive" diagnosis of cancer is communicated to the wrong OR.

Specifically pertaining to breast cancer frozen sections, it is not advisable to access surgical margin. Fatty tissue does not cut by using the cryostat machine and the margin assessment will be disrupted for permanent section. Certain surgeons request a pathologist to come to OR for gross intraoperatively to ink the cut specimen, to assess surgical margins for lumpectomy and mastectomy. Most lumpectomy specimens are assessed by radiology for surgical margins before the specimens are transferred to the pathology department. And therefore, the effort is duplicated if pathologist is cutting the specimen in the OR. Also, a pathologist can only accurately examine for the invasive carcinoma, which is palpable and visible, and not DCIS (in situ carcinoma). Both invasive and in-situ carcinomas must also be excised with clear surgical margin. And therefore, the intraoperative gross examination by a pathologist is not ideal.

The other situation for breast cancer cases where frozen section can be used, is for sentinel lymph node(s). The concept and the technique of the sentinel node will be discussed in a subsequent chapter. Surgeons are differing in their opinions to send frozen section examination for sentinel lymph node. Certain surgeons routinely submit a frozen section for sentinel lymph node, and others send only after a neoadjuvant chemotherapy setting. The role of frozen section in sentinel lymph node for breast cancer in the era of the ACOSOG Z0011 and IBCSG23-10 trials is rather clear, stating that it is not advisable. The guidelines recommend irradiation of lymph node, rather than completion axillary dissection with ≥4 axillary metastatic lymph nodes. And hence, there is no clear reason to freeze sentinel lymph node intraoperatively to decide whether to do completion axillary dissection or not. The studies above found frozen section has a low sensitivity in detecting smaller (micro) metastases with 19% false negativity. However, after neoadjuvant chemotherapy, sentinel lymph node frozen section is indicated with the understanding the false negative rates are pertinent, because a completion axillary dissection is done when intraoperative sentinel lymph node is positive with either micro- or macrometastatic carcinoma.

Chapter 8:
What is a permanent section, and how is it performed?

There are multiple steps to create a permanent section slide from the tissue a surgeon provides to pathology:

1. When the surgeon cuts out the diseased portion of the tissue from the patient, the specimen is labeled with the unique identification of the patient and delivered to pathology. We then accession the case with a unique surgical case number (S-21-20966). S stands for Surgical Specimen, 21 stands for the year 2021, and 20966 stands for the unique number for the specimen which means it is the 20966th specimen pathology received that year. Assigning a unique surgical number to the case, linking the specimen to the patient who had surgery, is "accessioning." To protect patient identification, the pathologist assigns this specific number which is not to be duplicated within the same year. We do this to protect patient confidentiality.

Because there are many people who work in a department of pathology, we do not want to spread news of a particular patient to the public. I have seen this occur. If the patient is a famous movie star, for instance, workers in a pathology department may recognize the name and spread gossip to co-workers or others, and eventually the media will become aware, with news vans swarming into the parking lots of hospitals and this is precisely why we generate the surgical number on each case. The specimen can be large (1,000 kg breast: 2.2 pounds) or a leg amputation weighing 20–30 pounds or more. When I receive such large permanent section specimens I am surprised by the warmth of the detached organ or body parts and always feel sad that the patient just lost a part of theirself. I have a deep respect for every specimen and empathize with the complex and tortuous pathway the patient went through, and emotional burdens they carry.

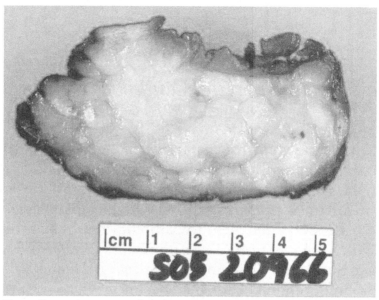

Breast lumpectomy cut in cross section. The surfaces are inked in multiple colors. Beneath the ruler, the surgical case is from 2005 and the unique number is 20966.

2. All specimens must be "fixed" before cutting by either the pathologist or pathology assistant (PA). The usual/routine fixative is 10% neutral buffer formaldehyde (formalin) which stops the decaying process. Once the body parts are detached from the blood supply, decaying process begins. Formalin is a chemical solution that fixes tissue to prevent degradation. A typical formalin fixation takes place overnight. For breast specimens, the minimum of 6 hours and the maximum of 72 hours (3 days) of fixation in formalin is required. The fixative soaks through the tissue at a constant rate, 1 mm per hour. So, if the tissue is thick, it requires a longer fixation time. For instance, breast tissue in mastectomy is large and fatty, requiring more time to fix. Interestingly, breast surgeons in particular want answers the quickest from the pathologist because their patients are most anxious. But to do a good job in pathology, the breast tissue must be fixed which takes time. Immunohistochemical stains will not provide accurate prognostic breast biomarkers if the breast tissue is not fixed well. A fast answer may not be the best answer in breast cases.

Anatomic pathology department working hours are typically 8:00 am to 5:00 pm. On weekdays, there is usually someone in the department to receive the specimens to fix in formalin even after hours in many academic centers. However, weekend specimens create a logistical issue. To prevent the decay, we store specimens in a specially designed refrigerator (set to 4 degrees Celsius). On Monday, the pathology staff will retrieve all specimens from the refrigerator and begin accessioning. This refrigerator can be situated in a designated area within pathology (usually in the clinical laboratory side since we require few if any weekend staff in anatomic pathology). Communication between clinical and anatomic pathology becomes critical in this scenario, and I witnessed a few unusual situations.

I was on call for the weekend and the clinical laboratory technician paged me to ask what she should do with a leg that was too heavy and too big to fit into the refrigerator on Saturday afternoon. I had to figure out this logistical problem and find a bigger refrigerator, then tell the PA on Monday whereabouts this leg can be found for them to accession. Remarkable questions arose. "Where is the leg?" and, "Which refrigerator is big enough to fit an exceptionally heavy and long leg?" This led to, "Can you ask someone to help me lift and carry the leg into the refrigerator, because I'm not too strong and it's bigger than I am." But to me, this was an urgent problem. I must find this leg on Monday to accession and properly handle and manage the tissue.

3. Once the specimen is fixed in formalin, a PA or pathologist must cut the specimen. Then, texture, colors, appearance, and sometimes even smell of the fresh specimens are described. This process is called "gross description." It is like describing who, when, where, how, and why in a matter-of-fact approach. During grossing, the breast tissue is weighed, measured in three dimensions in centimeters, and the surface is inked with different colors to visualize the tumor at the margins microscopically. Inking of the specimen becomes particularly important because the tumor should not be at or close to the inked margins, otherwise this means the patient retained tumor within their breast. The surgeon's objective is to cut out all the tumorous area, and this too is how we help the surgeon.

Pathologists often describe their findings in terms of food characteristics for reasons unknown to me, such as "cottage cheese" for necrotic and friable tissue. While it gives a clear picture in my head of the gross specimen appearance, I prefer to describe in non-food related terms such as cystic, friable, necrotic, bosselated, bulging, etc.

4. The tissue is then "bread-loafed," cutting it sequentially, maintaining the orientations. Next, each slice is cut into smaller sizes to be fitted into the standard size cassettes.

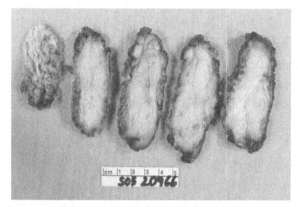

Breast tissue is cut serially (bread-loafed).

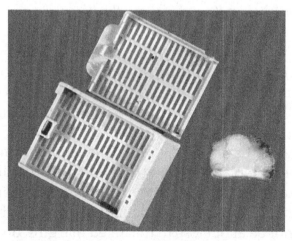

The length of a cassette (above) is 3.5 cm, the width 2.5 cm. The ideal amount of tissue is seen adjacent to the cassette and leaves room for the various solutions to penetrate well during machine processing.

5. For the routine breast specimen sample for lumpectomy (subtotal excision of the breast), total number of cassettes varies from 10–50. Each cassette of tissue will generate one slide. For mastectomy, it takes fewer cassettes (usually less than 20) because the surgical margins are usually negative. Then the specimen is sliced into multiple levels and cut sequentially into the cassettes. Tissue is cut during the day and processed overnight.

6. The cassettes are then loaded into a processing machine.

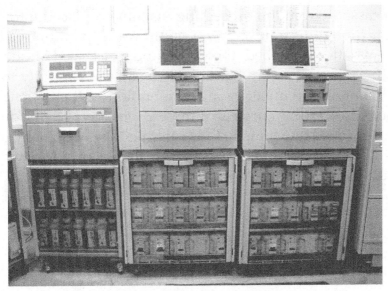

Three tissue processing machines are shown.

When the tissue is in the processing machine, it goes through at least nine different steps to fix the tissue with different chemical solutions. For the typical breast samples, due to the high fat content, it will take 9–12 hours for the processing machine to complete the fixation. Within each processing machine, there may be 100–300 patient samples in cassettes.

A rare event that occurred in one institution was due to cassette malfunction (the cassettes did not completely snap shut due to a rare cassette product defect). The next morning all the tissue fragments floated to the top of the solution. There was no way to know which tissue sample belonged to which patient. On this occasion, the hospital administration was involved and immediately began notifying all the affected patients that there would be no diagnosis from their tissue. The surgeons then had to remove additional tissue from patients, but for some patients, there was no residual tissue for the surgeon to resect and their samples were lost, and they would not know if they had malignancy. The magnitude of this extremely rare scenario demonstrates how important it is to maintain specimen integrity and identification in the pathology and surgery departments. Each step of the entire process is immensely important when handling a patient's tissue.

7. Each cassette from the processing machine is placed into position by a histology technician, who pours warm paraffin wax over a new cassette to embed the fixed and preserved tissue within paraffin. The technician handles each cassette carefully to embed and maintain the integrity and orientation of the patient sample without losing the surgical number. On average, the histology team receives a few hundred cassettes per day with many different patients' samples. It is of the utmost importance that we do not mix up the specimens from the different patients.

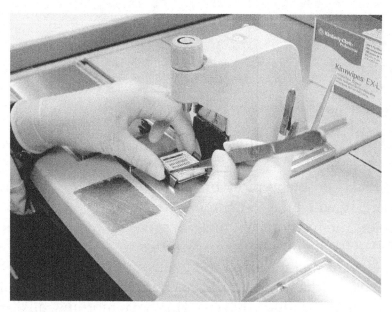

Embedding process by pouring warm wax.

8. Once the paraffin embedded tissue becomes colder after putting it on a block of ice, the cassette is placed in a microtome to cut thin

sections. It is important to cut the tissue deep enough into the paraffin to see the entire surface of the tissue section. The section thickness is usually 5–6 microns.

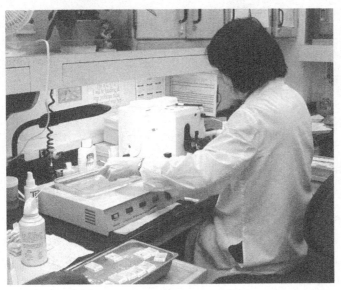

A histotechnician cutting formalin fixed paraffin embedded tissue after cooling with ice.

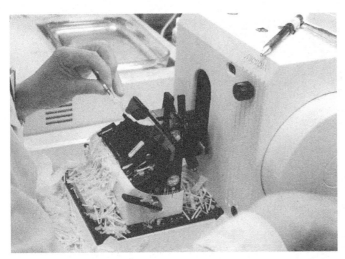

The ribbons of tissue are carefully plucked away and placed on the water bath to spread out all the wrinkling of the tissue.

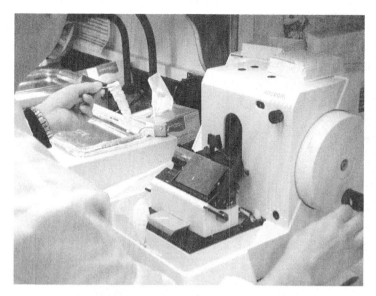

9. Once the tissue is evenly spread out, the technician picks up the best tissue with a glass slide. It is important to change the water bath constantly and between every case. This prevents cross contamination of different patient samples. The tissue is now out, on the glass slide and the technician labels each slide with the case and slide numbers.

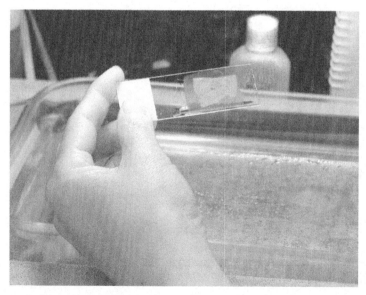

From the water bath, each tissue is picked up onto the glass slide. The surgical case number is written by the histotechnician.

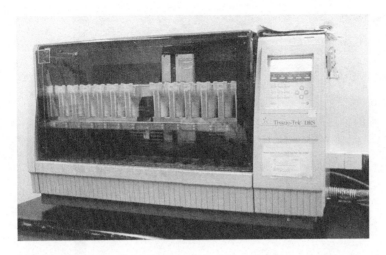

10. The slides then go into the automated H&E stain machine for staining. See above. This process will take an average of 2–3 hours. The work is batched to stain hundreds of slides from different patient samples.

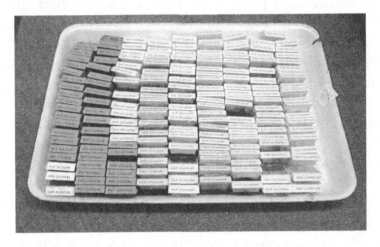

Assorted colors of cassettes can be used to prioritize the RUSH cases, routine cases, or breast cases (which generally take longer time to process).

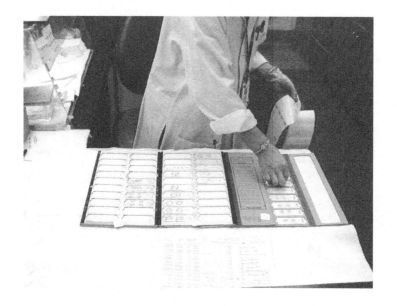

11. Once the automated H&E stain machine work is completed, the histology technicians place the labels on the finished slides. The slides are lined up on flats and delivered to pathologists for slides to be read. Histology technicians usually start their work in the middle of the night, 2:00 am to 4:00 am, so that all the slides are prepared to be read by the pathologists in the morning, often at 8:00 am. On a routine day, a pathologist can read 50–100 patient samples, and each sample may contain one to more than 50 slides. There is usually one sample per patient, but sometimes 2–20 tissue samples per case, each with multiple slides.

12. After reviewing slides of each patient's samples under the microscope, the pathologist generates their pathology report. It usually takes about one or more hours to look at a larger breast case such as lumpectomy or mastectomy with lymph nodes dissection. For a small needle biopsy specimen, it will take 5–20 minutes to arrive at a conclusion and identify and name the disease and generate the final diagnosis. Most pathologists dictate the final diagnosis to save time because talking is faster than typing. Typically, a pathologist spends an entire day to review their cases under the microscope and dictate the final diagnoses, sometimes dictating over 100 cases a day depending on the practice setting.

A typical pathology report will have the patient's name, medical record (identification number), the surgical number, the date of procedure, the surgeon's name and or requesting doctor's name, institution name, the name of the pathologist who generated the report, their final diagnosis, their microscopic examination, gross examination, and possibly additional ancillary tests such as immunohistochemical stains, cytogenetic studies, etc., and a synoptic CAP report if the diagnosis is malignant based on CAP guidelines and requirements and the date of the pathologist's sign out. Chapter 11 provides more details. An addendum report following the original report in the breast cancer cases includes the status of estrogen, progesterone receptors (ER, PR), Her-2/*neu* and Ki-67 for predictive and prognostic indicators.

13. After the pathologist's sign out, the report is entered into the hospital electronic medical record (EMR), so that any medical professional caring for the patient will be able to access the pathologist's findings, which we name FINAL DIAGNOSIS. No other medical profession except pathologists can generate the "final diagnosis." Rendering of the final diagnosis is the most important first step for the patient to receive appropriate care and treatment. Without the final diagnosis by a pathologist, no clinician—including surgeon—can help the patient. As one may conclude, the necessary fixation time, overnight machine processing, handling time by the histotechnician, and the pathologist's time to read the tissue slides all results in a minimum of 48 hours to generate a final diagnosis for a routine large specimen from the patient. If the case is unusual or challenging, additional ancillary tests take at least one more day, as in the case of the immunohistochemical stains, or even weeks, for cytogenetic tests. The pathologist must review all the ancillary test results and then put together the final diagnostic findings. A pathologist sometimes asks colleagues to read out the slides to gather further thoughts. This is defined as "internal departmental consultation." It is not unusual to take a week to sort things out to generate a final report from pathology. If the case is extraordinarily difficult, or there is no unanimous agreement between benign or malignancy in the diagnosis among the internal departmental pathologists, the case is sent to an outside institution for the "expert consultation"

from well-known pathologists in the specific field. The department carefully packages the case slides and pathology report for overnight delivery. One or two weeks is typical turn-around-time for expert consultation results.

It is critically important the integrity of a specific patient sample retains its identity tied to the patient throughout these multiple steps; from the time of removal of tissue from the operation room to a pathologist signing out the case and inputting the final diagnosis into the electronic medical record. Each day, a pathologist can receive over 100 surgical cases from outpatient surgical centers, internal hospital main operation rooms, and satellite surgical offices. Maintaining integrity in logistical tissue movement and tracking is essential and allows for accurately reading and diagnosing each case so that every patient is provided the correct diagnosis. This requires tremendous mechanical system reliance, documentation, and quality control. Any mistake from one person can have detrimental effects by mismatch of patient samples.

Chapter 9:
Different types of biopsies for breast cancers

1. **Fine needle aspiration (FNA):** This procedure is generally considered a safe procedure and minimally invasive. Complications are infrequent. There is no pre-procedural diet or any limitations in drinking fluids. Anesthesia is not needed. At times, local topical spray to numb the area may be used. FNA is usually performed by cytopathologists. Other physicians such as clinicians and radiologists can also perform FNA procedures. The needle bore sizes are 27, 25 and 23 gauge, and the appropriate gauge needle is inserted into an FNA gun (holder). The needle extracts cells from the mass which are then expressed directly onto the slide and smeared. The specimens are not tissue fragments but individual cells on the slide, and usually signed out by the cytopathologists. The slides are then stained with Papanicolaou or May-Grunwald-Giemsa (MGG) stains (not routinely with Hematoxylin and Eosin as in the surgical specimens). Papanicolaou stain is an excellent stain for visualizing the nuclear features, and MGG stain is excellent for cytoplasmic features. There are multiple limitations using FNA for breast cancer. First, FNA cannot easily distinguish invasive breast carcinoma from ductal carcinoma in situ (DCIS) which is a precursor lesion to invasive carcinoma. Both DCIS and invasive carcinoma cells are malignant by FNA. Another limitation is the technical requirements for breast prognostic markers (ER, PR and Her-2/*neu*) are not consistent, and not ideal. CAP guidelines for the breast prognostic markers require 10% formalin paraffin embedded tissue. FNA slides are fixed in alcohol, not 10% formalin and hence it is preferred not to have confirmatory studies in ER, PR and Her-2/*neu*. However, cell blocks can be made from needle washings and placed in 10% formalin to achieve this purpose.

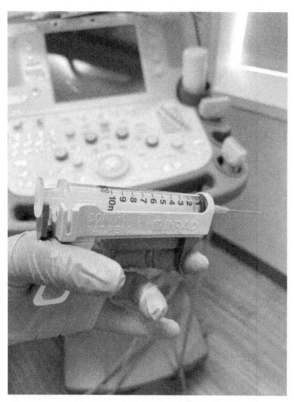

Image provided by Dr. Neda Moatamed, FNA Director from UCLA. She is holding the FNA gun with 10 ml syringe and 25 gauge needle. Ultrasound machine shown in background.

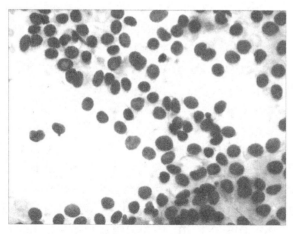

FNA yields individual cells without architectural arrangement of tissue. This is an example of papillary thyroid carcinoma from a young female patient's sample from the thyroid.

2. **Core needle biopsy (CNB):** Core needle is a larger bore needle which will yield a tissue fragment. A core biopsy is routinely done at the radiology setting, assisted by ultrasound (US), stereotactic or MR image-guided methods. US-guided biopsy is done when there is a mass lesion. Stereotactic biopsy is done when there is calcification detected by mammogram. MRI-guided biopsy is done when the lesion is seen by MRI. A core needle biopsy is the preferred type of biopsy if breast cancer is suspected because the pathologist can see the architectural pattern as well as cytology of the cancer cells in relationship with the background tissue to distinguish invasive carcinoma and DCIS. The breast prognostic biomarker studies are limited to only ER and PR for DCIS. Full breast prognostic studies are done for invasive breast cancer such as ER, PR, and Her-2/*neu* to determine whether the patient may need presurgical neoadjuvant chemotherapy before the definitive surgical excision to shrink the tumor size before proceeding with lumpectomy rather than mastectomy.

Her-2/*neu* positive and triple negative (ER, PR and Her-2/*neu* negative) breast tumors are known to be more aggressive subtypes of tumors, and neoadjuvant chemotherapy is routinely given. Since core needle biopsy is an ideal specimen type for the breast prognostic studies, it is the preferred method in diagnosing breast cancer.

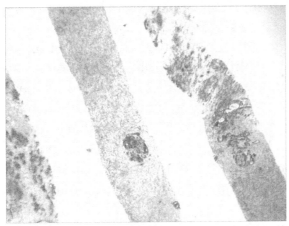

An example of core needle biopsy where three tissue fragments are seen from this image. Each core has normal breast ducts, and infiltrating breast cancer in a background of fibrosis.

3. **Incisional biopsy versus excisional biopsy:** Incisional biopsy is to remove a piece of tissue from a lesion or mass, but not the entire lesion, for testing and determining the cancer type. Incisional biopsy is a larger piece than core needle biopsy and usually performed by a surgeon. Incisional biopsy is for diagnostic purpose without surgical margin, whereas excisional biopsy is not just for diagnostic purpose but also to evaluate surgical margin.

   The terminology of excisional biopsy is the same as lumpectomy. A term of excisional biopsy is preferred in which the whole lesion or mass is removed and tested. In pathology as well as in surgery, this term is preferred when the lesion is benign, such as fibroadenoma. For benign lesions, surgical margin assessment is often not accessed. The term lumpectomy is used when the lesion is malignant, either DCIS or invasive breast carcinoma. For the malignant lesions, surgical margin assessment must be reported.

4. **Lumpectomy and mastectomy:** *Lumpectomy* is a surgery to remove cancerous breast tissue along with a rim of normal tissue surrounding it with clear surgical margin. Lumpectomy synonym is a wide local excision, segmentectomy, quadrantectomy, or partial mastectomy. Lumpectomy can be done with or without wire guided localization. Wire localization is done predominantly when the calcifications are suspicious for precancerous condition such as DCIS. Wire localization is done by a radiologist and lumpectomy is done by a surgeon.

   Mastectomy is a surgery to remove the whole breast including the nipple and areolar complex. Simple mastectomy and total mastectomy are synonymous. Radical mastectomy has become mostly obsolete, and is a surgery to remove the whole breast, chest wall including pectoralis muscle, and axillary lymph node dissections. Modified radical mastectomy is a surgery to remove the whole breast, axillary lymph nodes and fascia superficial to the chest wall pectoral muscle and is now more common.

5. **Axillary sentinel lymph node biopsy:** Sentinel lymph node is a first draining lymph node from the cancerous breast. It is usually located at the axillary arm pit area from the same side of the cancerous breast but at times, it can be located at the middle (thorax) or even rarely the opposite axillary side. Sentinel lymph

node is detected either or both by the blue dye method and/or radioactive tracer method which is injected prior to the surgery. The first lymph node to drain the dye and/or tracer is called sentinel lymph node. At times, there are multiple sentinel lymph nodes. Removal of sentinel lymph node(s) is/(are) a less invasive and morbid surgery than a full axillary dissection. The latter surgery includes risk of bleeding, infection, nerve injury, lymphedema, and loss of range of motion of arm and shoulder.

6. **Axillary lymph node dissection:** This is a procedure also called lymphadenectomy to remove the entire arm pit lymph nodes and ranges from 10–40 lymph nodes. On average it is a little less than 20. The risk of complications is more common than sentinel lymph node biopsy procedure. A thorough search for the axillary lymph nodes is prudent by the pathologist or PA. A minimum of ten lymph nodes is required for the full axillary dissection. If there are less than ten lymph nodes, then, the entire fat tissue is submitted to look for small lymph nodes within the fat.

7. **Skin punch biopsy:** A punch biopsy of the breast takes a sample of the skin and underlying dermis tissue. A punch biopsy is commonly used if the lesion is evident from superficial surface of the skin. The most common condition of the skin punch biopsy is for the pigmented lesion such as to rule out melanoma. For breast disease, a punch biopsy is used when *Paget's disease* and/or inflammatory breast cancer is present, or mass lesion directly underneath the skin, skin discoloration, eczema, or inflamed appearance. *Paget's disease* is when ductal carcinoma in situ and/or invasive breast cancer cells are found within the epidermis. An inflammatory breast cancer diagnosis is confirmed by having both clinical and pathologic changes meeting the diagnostic criteria; clinically the breast skin changes include redness, warmth, swelling, skin thickening, orange peel appearance, and pathologically the presence of superficial dermal lymph-vascular invasion.

Chapter 10:
Whose property are the slides and blocks from pathology?

I have seen patients demand their slides and blocks be sent to whoever and wherever they want, thinking the items belong to them. It is true that the tissue came from the patient's sample, but the slides and tissue blocks are protected and retained by the original pathology department from the hospital or commercial laboratory. Technically, once detached from the body, the excised specimens no longer belong to the patient. Pathology departments are the recognized legal caretakers of these tissues, and there are no specific state or federal rules regarding ownership of diagnostic tissue blocks.

The Joint Commission (TJC) and the College of American Pathologists (CAP) also have their own guidelines and recommendations, aside from state laws for maintaining the slides and tissue blocks. This also ensures their availability for future study should new testing or treatments for the patient's disease be developed. The pathology departments are legal guardians to preserve and protect the tissue blocks and slides. Recut slides are easily made from the tissue block, but the tissue block itself cannot be replaced once lost. If blocks must be moved outside the original facility for a medical or legal reason, or for additional genetic testing per a clinician or patient request, the pathology department should carefully document the tissue block location, movement, including receipt of all materials by the recipients, date, and condition of the returned blocks.

All tissues procured by a surgeon during a procedure must be transferred directly to the pathology department without any interference. I have seen aggressive researchers take pieces of tissue from the operation room for their research, sometimes without pathology knowledge, which violates the tissue integrity for the diagnostic purposes in terms of the size of the tumor (which affects T-stage of the tumor) and the surgical margins. Only exception to this rule should be when the patient has consented to have research specimens collected (not for diagnostic purpose), and the researchers have Institutional

Review Boards (IRB) approval from their institution for a specific research project.

Increasingly, tissues from pathology departments are being requested for research purposes, especially in the current era of precision medicine. There are no prohibitions on the use of these tissues in biomedical research, provided that the pathology department follows state laws regarding maintenance of these blocks, ensures diagnostic tissues remain available, and abide by federal research regulations and institutional policies. For the human-subjects research, the IRB must prospectively review it to ensure compliance with federal research regulations. Federal policies on human research are codified in the *Code of Federal Regulations (45 CFR part 46, Subpart A*—also known as the *Common Rule*) and in the *Health Insurance Portability and Accountability Act (HIPAA)* passed in 1996. Pathology departments can release the tissue block only after the IRB approval, IRB exemption, or a letter from the IRB stating IRB approval is not required prior to distributing blocks or sections from diagnostic tissue blocks for research.

The pathologist is the silent protector and legal caretaker for the patients and work on their behalf behind the scenes. Every tissue block will have DNA from the patient. And it is the pathologist who protects the patient's tissue.

III. The diagnosis

Chapter 11:
What is in the pathology report and what does it mean?

A typical core needle biopsy for the breast cancer pathology report needs to have the following information.

1. Institution name.
2. Name of the patient.
3. Patient's medical number.
4. Patient's birthdate.
5. Procedure date.
6. Ordering physician's name (usually the radiologist's name who is performing the core biopsy with the imaging modality methods; stereotactic for microcalcifications or asymmetry, ultrasound for mass lesion or Magnetic Resonance Imaging (MRI) for enhancing lesion or asymmetry).
7. Attending/Treating physician's name or copy lists of other physician's names. (This is when the patient has been seen by other doctors including the previous surgeons and oncologists within the same institution).
8. Date of receipt from pathology.
    The procedure date and pathology accession date may be different, especially late afternoon or weekend procedures. The core needle biopsy is placed in formalin solution and hence it generally would not have any negative impact for the specimen quality and preservation.
9. Organ site. (Breast, axillary lymph node, etc.)
10. Laterality. (Left or right)
11. Procedure name. (Stereotactic, US or MRI)

12. Surgical number. (Unique pathology number)
13. Final diagnosis lists: (Example given is for a cancer case)
    a. Invasive ductal carcinoma, Grade 1, 2 or 3.
    b. Modified Bloom and Richardson score 3-5 (grade 1), 6-7 (grade 2), 8-9 (grade 3) of 9.
       i.   Tubule formation grade 1, 2 or 3.
       ii. Nuclear pleomorphism grade 1, 2 or 3.
       iii. Mitotic count grade 1, 2 or 3.
    c. Ductal carcinoma in situ. (DCIS)
       i.   Nuclear grade 1, 2 or 3. (Or low, intermediate, or high)
       ii. Presence or absence of central/comedo necrosis.
       iii. Architectural pattern: solid, cribriform, comedo types etc.
    d. Presence or absence of lymph-vascular invasion.
    e. Presence or absence of microcalcifications; if present, then associated with what lesion(s).
    f. Breast prognostic biomarkers:
       i.   Estrogen Receptor (ER) in percentage positivity (0–100%) and intensity (1+ to 3+).
       ii. Progesterone Receptor (PR) in percentage positivity (0–100%) and intensity (1+ to 3+).
       iii. Her-2/*neu*: Immunohistochemical (IHC) stain (score 0, 1+, 2+ or 3+) with description not overexpressed, indeterminate, or overexpressed.
       iv. Her-2/*neu* by in situ hybridization. (Routinely, Fluorescent In-Situ Hybridization (FISH) with ratio of Her-2 to CEP 17 and Her-2 copy number in numerical number and the description stating not amplified, indeterminate, or amplified).
            Certain pathology laboratories perform FISH only when Her-2/*neu* by IHC stain shows a score of 2+ which is indeterminate.
       v.   Ki-67 in percentage. (Proliferative index which is related to mitotic count). Certain pathology laboratories do not routinely perform Ki-67.
    g. Any additional comments from pathologist to clinicians.
    h. Microscopic examination descriptions.

Minimal microscopic description is "performed," which means the slide is made and then reviewed by the pathologist.

i. Gross examination descriptions.
    This section describes what the specimen looked like such as number of cores, the measurement of the cores, and the appearance if unique. This section also needs to include how many cassettes are submitted, with the initials of the pathologist, PA, or technician who handled the gross specimen.
j. Pathologist's signature. (This is the original pathologist's name who prepared the report and reviewed the slides).
k. Date and time of the final diagnosis pathology report.
l. CLIA number with CLIA Director's name. (Pathology Laboratory Director for the group).
m. Transcriptionist initials if there is a transcriptionist.

For the core needle biopsy, the surgical margins, size of the tumors for both invasive and DCIS may not be included. Other institutions may include the size of invasive carcinoma from the core needle biopsy stating "at least ___ cm from the limited sample." Any additional immunohistochemical stains for diagnostic purpose can be added in the microscopic section or immunohistochemical stain section below the final diagnosis with results either positive or negative, and interpretation. For example, p63 stain is positive and the interpretation is "supportive of DCIS and no invasive carcinoma."

For the typical excisional biopsy report a small number of additional items in the final diagnosis should be included:
1. Size of invasive carcinoma/tumor in centimeters.
2. Size of DCIS or volume of DCIS including whether extensive intraductal component (EIC) is present or absent.
3. Surgical margins: positive or negative in terms of invasive carcinoma and DCIS.
4. Any other findings such as presence of biopsy site changes, micro clip(s) and other benign or interesting lesions in the breast, aside from the tumor.

5. Nipple/skin. If present, descriptions whether dermal lymphovascular invasion and/or Paget's disease is present or absent.
6. Skeletal muscle. Whether present or absent and whether the tumor is seen or not.
7. *American Joint Committee on Cancer (AJCC) Tumor Node Metastasis (TNM) stage.*
8. Oncotype Dx Recurrence score. (This is not always present in the pathology report and seen only in the addendum report when the clinician orders Oncotype Dx). It is a genomic-based, individualized risk assessment for early-stage invasive breast cancer in ER positive, Her-2/*neu* negative and node-negative and sometimes up to 3 lymph nodes positive, Polymerase Chain Reaction (PCR) test to determine whether adjuvant chemotherapy is needed or not in addition to anti-hormonal therapy. Her-2/*neu* positive or triple negative breast cancer regardless of lymph node metastasis will require adjuvant or neoadjuvant chemotherapy and therefore no need to send for Oncotype Dx.

For the lymph node report, the following items need to be stated:
1. How many sentinel lymph node(s) are identified.
2. How many total lymph nodes are identified.
3. How many lymph node(s) is(are) positive for metastatic carcinoma.
4. If metastatic carcinoma is present, classify as isolated tumor cells (ITC), micrometastatic or macrometastatic carcinoma.
5. If there is a metastatic carcinoma in the lymph node, then additional information must be further characterized:
   a. Size of maximum dimension of the metastatic carcinoma (in millimeter or centimeter).
   b. Extranodal extension present or absent. For example,
      - Two out of eleven lymph nodes are positive for macrometastatic carcinoma (2/11).
      - Maximum linear dimension of metastatic carcinoma measures 2.6 mm.
      - Extranodal extension present measuring 1.0 mm.

What is the meaning of all the words in a pathology report and what is the significance?

1. *Type of breast cancer:* There are numerous variants of breast cancers. The most common type is invasive ductal carcinoma (85–90%). The second most common type is invasive lobular carcinoma (approximately 10%). Other types of invasive carcinomas include cribriform, tubular, mucinous, metaplastic (adenosquamous, squamous, spindle), medullary, papillary, lipid-rich, glycogen rich, micropapillary, secretory, acinar cell, mucoepidermoid, adenoid cystic, tall cell with reversed polarity, neuroendocrine tumor, neuroendocrine carcinoma.

2. *Modified Bloom and Richardson scores and grade*: There are three items to score between 1–3; nuclear pleomorphism, mitotic count and tubular/glandular pattern. Grade 3 has poor prognosis and grade 1 has better prognosis.

3. *Ductal carcinoma in situ (DCIS)* is a precursor lesion to invasive breast cancer. There are numerous variants and patterns of DCIS. Type, grade, presence or absence of central necrosis should be included in the pathology report. The Comedo type has the worst prognosis which has high grade (grade 3) and presence of central necrosis. The most common DCIS are cribriform and solid pattern. Grade 1 DCIS has better prognosis than grade 3 DCIS.

4. Since mammogram detects *calcifications* in the breast by radiologist, it is important to address which lesion is associated with microcalcifications in a pathology report. If microcalcification is associated with DCIS, then, surgeons will map out the amount of tissue to be removed by wire localization.

5. *Size of invasive carcinoma and DCIS:* Bigger the cancer size, the worst prognosis. Size of the tumor is reported as T-stage.

6. *Extensive intraductal component (EIC):* The amount of DCIS greater than 25–30% from the tissue removed in association of invasive breast cancer has a predictive value on whether the tissue remained in the patient may have residual disease. EIC absent has better prognosis. EIC present means it is most likely that the patient will have residual DCIS or invasive carcinoma in the breast tissue that was not removed. The presence of EIC is considered to be an important risk factor for local recurrence in lumpectomy.

7. *Surgical margins* are reported for both invasive carcinoma and DCIS. All lumpectomy and mastectomy specimens are inked before cutting to study whether the surgeon has removed all the disease components. According to *NCCN guidelines,* no ink on

tumor suffices in breast cancer treatment *(https://www.nccn.org)*. The pathology report, according to CAP guidelines, should record the distance from all six margins for invasive carcinoma and DCIS in closest centimeters. Greater than or equal to 1.0 cm (10 mm) is considered widely excised margin.

8. *Lymph-vascular invasion (LVI):* Within the breast tissue, there are vascular and lymphatic structures. If invasive breast cancer cells are seen within these structures, it is a worse prognosis, and the risk of lymph node metastasis increases.

9. *Estrogen and Progesterone receptors status* has both prognostic and predictive values. ER and PR positive tumors have better prognosis, and it is predictive that anti-estrogen therapy such as Tamoxifen and Aromatase inhibitor drugs will be beneficial to prevent recurrence and metastasis. ER and PR status are done for both DCIS and invasive carcinoma. Her-2/*neu* and Ki-67 are added for invasive carcinoma. (DCIS cases do not routinely report Her-2/*neu* and Ki-67).

10. *Her-2/neu status* has both prognostic and predictive values. Her-2/*neu* positive breast cancer has a poor prognosis, and it is predictive that anti-Her2 therapy will be beneficial to prevent recurrence and metastasis. It is important to have Her-2/*neu* study done by two methods, in my opinion: Immunohistochemical staining and the ISH method. Triple negative breast cancers are defined by ER, PR, and Her-2/*neu* negative tumors. Triple negative breast cancer has no targetable and predictive therapeutic regimens and hence, the worst type of breast cancer to have. Recently a Phase 3 trial involving patients with Her2-low (score of 1+ or 2+) metastatic breast cancer with negative on in situ hybridization who received anti-Her2 therapy resulted in significantly longer progression-free and overall survival rate. Hence, it is important to accurately score IHC Her2 staining. *(NEJM DOI: 10.1056/NEJMoa2203690)*

11. *Ki-67 status:* Higher Ki-67 is related to cell proliferation index and has a poor prognosis. Ki-67 of less than 10% has best prognosis and is commonly related to grade 1 invasive breast carcinoma.

12. *Lymph node metastasis* is related to N-stage in the pathology report. It has a poor prognosis if lymph node shows metastatic carcinoma. The size of the metastatic disease in the lymph node is divided as follows:

a. *Isolated tumor cells (ITC)*: Very small number of metastatic tumor cells often detected only by IHC stains. When ITC is present, the lymph node is designated to be N0 (i+) and will not count as a positive lymph node.
b. *Micrometastasis*: Metastatic tumor measures greater than 0.2 mm to less than or equal to 2 mm.
c. *Macrometastasis*: Metastatic tumor measures greater than 2 mm. Micro and macrometastatic tumors count as a positive lymph node.
d. *Extranodal extension (ENE)* is when tumor cells are seen beyond the lymph node structure and into fat tissue surrounding the lymph node. If present, the prognosis is worse. It is subdivided into >2 mm or ≤ 2 mm.

13. *Genomic tests:* There are multiple available genomic tests for breast cancers. MammaPrint made by Agendia, Breast Cancer Index test, EndoPredict test, Prosigna Breast Cancer Prognostic Gene Signature Assay (PAM 50), and Oncotype Dx. Oncotype Dx is the most prevalent test breast oncologists order and is further explained below.

Oncotype test:
The oncologists can order this test which is one of the genomic tests to navigate whether a patient needs chemotherapy along with hormonal therapy. According to the manufacturer of this test, the indication for this test is for early-stage breast cancer (T1 or T2; Stage 1-IIIa) with node negative breast cancer. Most clinicians will not send stage IIIa disease out for oncotype testing and will treat with chemotherapy. However, some oncologists order this test even with T3 and with node positive tumors. The Oncotype Dx generates a Recurrence Score (RS), a score of 0–100 based on 21 specific genes in the breast tumor tissue (usually from excision and not core needle biopsy samples). RS scores are divided into low, intermediate, and high. Low RS generally do not have any benefit for chemotherapy and high RS generally means the patient needs chemotherapy. For the intermediate RS, the TAILORx clinical trial enrolled 10,273 patients over 1,000 sites to understand whether chemotherapy may benefit along with hormonal therapy. Most patients with RS score of 0–25 did not benefit from additional

chemotherapy whereas RS score of 26–100 showed significant benefit by adding chemotherapy.

As one can see, it is the pathologist's report that guides the treatment and further management by providing the findings from each patient's breast cancer. One can argue the pathology is the most important aspect of how the patient with breast cancer can be treated. Based on the pathologic findings, algorithm as to how the patient will be treated are spelled out. And hence, it is the pathologists who can generate "The Final Diagnosis." No other fields of medicine can use this term of final diagnosis. They can use "differential diagnosis" or "probable diagnosis."

Radiologists are also in the field of providing diagnostic tests and can provide their findings and best prediction what the lesion will turn out to be. One of my radiology colleagues said, "When I state BI-RADS 5, this means I am betting my house that it will turn out to be a cancer," and also added, "my house is not cheap!" BI-RADS stands for Breast Imaging-Reporting and Data System. It provides standardized assessment, organization of reports, and classifications for breast images including mammography, ultrasound, and MRI. Developed by the American College of Radiology, all breast radiologists use this lexicon which has become a uniform language in fields of breast cancer.

While the radiologist was not wrong in his bet when he signed out the BI-RADS 5, it was still his best guess and only a pathologist can confirm the presence of breast cancer. It is ironic the pathologist—the unseen doctor—is behind curtains, not visible to patients, yet perhaps the most powerful doctor who can provide the final diagnosis which will affect the entire downstream management and treatment for the patient.

Time required for pathology reports:
- Routine pathology reports take 1–7 days to generate. The core needle biopsy report will take 1–3 days after the procedure. The excisional biopsy (lumpectomy and mastectomy) report will take longer than core needle biopsy (2–7 days) due to longer fixation time, many more slides and filling out the synoptic report.
- Immunohistochemistry test takes one additional day. And hence, breast biomarkers are routinely reported as *addendum diagnosis #1.*

- Any ISH test, whether it is FISH, CISH or DISH tests for Her-2/*neu* gene amplification and may take 1–7 additional day(s). And therefore, ISH results are reported as *addendum report #2*.
- Oncotype DX tests are ordered by oncologic colleagues after all the results are available to delineate whether adding chemotherapy will be beneficial on an individual patient situation. The request for Oncotype test is sent out and the result will take additional 1–2 weeks. At some institutions, this result will be added as addendum report #3. So, it is not unusual to have three additional addendum reports in one breast cancer case.

For the core needle biopsy pathology report, it is usually 3–5 pages and for the lumpectomy or mastectomy report, it is usually an 8–10 pages per patient case. For the lumpectomy or mastectomy for DCIS and invasive breast cancer, a synoptic report must be included according to CAP guidelines.

Positions of a pathology report and for mastectomy, below.

Surgical Pathology Report

DIAGNOSIS:
A) BREAST, RIGHT (TOTAL MASTECTOMY):
- INVASIVE DUCTAL CARCINOMA:
  - MODIFIED SBR SCORE: 8/9 (GRADE 3):
    - TUBULAR DIFFERENTIATION: 3/3
    - NUCLEAR PLEOMORPHISM: 2/3
    - MITOTIC ACTIVITY: 3/3
- SIZE OF INVASIVE CARCINOMA: 2.3 CM.
- ASSOCIATED DUCTAL CARCINOMA IN-SITU (DCIS).
  - NUCLEAR GRADE: INTERMEDIATE
  - ARCHITECTURE: SOLID AND CRIBRIFORM
  - NECROSIS: PRESENT
- EXTENSIVE INTRADUCTAL COMPONENT: PRESENT (DCIS IS ESTIMATED TO BE 90% OF TUMOR VOLUME, SPANNING 7.0 CM)
- SURGICAL MARGINS:
  - ALL MARGINS APPEAR NEGATIVE FOR TUMOR.
- MICROCALCIFICATIONS PRESENT IN ASSOCIATION WITH BENIGN BREAST DUCTS, DCIS AND FIBROUS STROMA.
- LYMPH-VASCULAR INVASION: NOT IDENTIFIED
- BACKGROUND BREAST TISSUE WITH BIOPSY SITE CHANGES.
- SKIN/NIPPLE: NO DERMAL LYMPHATIC INVASION OR PAGET'S DISEASE SEEN
- ONE AXILLARY LYMPH NODE, NEGATIVE FOR METASTATIC CARCINOMA (0/1).
- TNM STAGE (AJCC 8TH ED): T2 N0 (sn)

B. RIGHT AXILLARY SENTINEL LYMPH NODE (BIOPSY):
- ONE LYMPH NODE NEGATIVE FOR METASTATIC CARCINOMA (0/1) (SEE

Portion of an addendum report, below.

Addendum Report

Addendum Discussion
#1

RESULTS OF BREAST BIOMARKERS TESTING

BREAST, RIGHT (TOTAL MASTECTOMY)

Immunohistochemical stains performed on formalin-fixed paraffin-embedded sections from block A13 and reviewed with the corresponding H&E section demonstrate the following results:

Estrogen Receptor (Ventana clone SP1): >95% of the neoplastic nuclei exhibit nuclear positivity and average strong intensity of staining consistent with a **POSITIVE** result.

Progesterone Receptor (Dako clone 1294): 70% of the neoplastic nuclei exhibit nuclear positivity and average moderate intensity of staining consistent with a **POSITIVE** result.

HER2: (Ventana clone 4B5): Membrane staining that is incomplete and faint/barely perceptible within </=10% of tumor cells consistent with a **NEGATIVE** result (SCORE 0).

p53: (Ventana clone DO7): Less than 5% of the neoplastic nuclei are positive **(favorable)**.

Ki-67: (Ventana clone 30-9): Greater than 40% of the neoplastic nuclei are positive **(unfavorable)**.

Cold ischemia and formalin fixation times meet requirements specified in latest version of the ASCO/CAP guidelines

The results by immunohistochemical method for hormone receptor testing are reported following the most recent CAP-ASCO guidelines using FDA approved commercially available tests by the above specified vendors. ER and PR are semi-quantitated and considered positive if ≥1% of tumor cells exhibit nuclear staining with average intensity graded as weak, moderate, and/or strong. HER2 is scored based on extent of membrane positivity from 0-3+. A HER2 score of 0 is given for absent membrane staining or faint incomplete

Chapter 12:
How does a pathologist stage each breast cancer?

There are five stages of breast cancer:

Stage 0

Cancer cells are not in invasive state, and this is called in situ. These can be ductal carcinoma in situ (DCIS) lobular carcinoma in situ (LCIS) or Paget's disease in nipple without invasive component underneath the breast. Currently, LCIS is removed from the stage in the AJCC 8th ed. (Tis, N0, M0)

Stage 1

Cancer is in invasive state but is contained only in the breast, subdivided into 1A and 1B.

1A is when invasive breast cancer tumor size is up to 2 cm and the cancer has not spread outside the breast. (T1, N0, M0)

1B is when invasive breast cancer tumor size is no larger than 2 cm and there are small groups of cancer cells (0.2 mm to 2 mm) in the same side armpit lymph node, and we call this ipsilateral axillary lymph node the axillary lymph node.

1B also includes when there is no tumor in the breast, but small groups of cancer cells found in the axillary lymph node, again measuring 0.2 mm to 2 mm. (T0 or T1, N1mi, M0)

Stage 2

This is subdivided into IIA and IIB.

IIA is when the tumor size is not bigger than 2 cm but spread to the axillary lymph node and this metastasis measures greater than 2 mm, or no tumor found in the breast, but the axillary lymph node metastasis is greater than 2 mm in 1–3 lymph node(s), or the tumor size is greater than 2 cm but less than 5 cm without the axillary lymph node metastasis. (T0, N1, M0/T1, N1, M0/T2, N0, M0)

IIB is a tumor larger than 2 cm, but less than 5 cm and small groups of metastases are found in the axillary lymph node, or the tumor is 2–5 cm in size and has spread to 1–3 axillary lymph nodes, or the tumor size is greater than 5 cm without spread to the axillary lymph node. (T2, N1, M0/T3, N0, M0)

Stage 3

This is subdivided into IIIA, IIIB and IIIC.

IIIA is when the tumor in any size with 4–9 axillary lymph node metastases or bone metastasis, or the tumor size greater than 5 cm with axillary lymph node containing small groups of metastases or the tumor size greater than 5 cm with greater than 2 mm in 1–3 axillary lymph nodes or bone metastasis. (T0, T1, T2 or T3, N2, M0/T3, N1, M0)

IIIB is when the tumor size in any size but has spread to the chest wall and/or skin of the breast with clinical evidence of swelling or ulcer or spread into more than 9 axillary lymph nodes. (T4, N0, N1, N2, M0)

IIIC is when there is no sign of breast cancer or any size of breast cancer but spread into the chest wall and/or skin or metastasis in more than 10 axillary lymph nodes or metastasis into the collar bones. (Any T, N3, M0)

Stage 4

This is when invasive breast cancer has spread beyond the breast and axillary lymph nodes to other organs of the body. This is the most advanced stage of the cancer. (Any T, any N, M1)

What is a TNM stage?

TNM stage is used for all cancers by pathologists. T-stands for tumor size, N-stands for lymph node and M-stands for metastasis. Since 1959, the *American Joint Committee of Cancer (AJCC)* has published this "universal language" of cancer. Most recently, pathologists are using the *8th Edition*.

For breast cancers, T-stages are categorized as the following:

Primary Tumor (Invasive Carcinoma) (pT)

pTX:	Primary tumor cannot be assessed
pT0:	No evidence of primary tumor
pTis (DCIS):	Ductal carcinoma in situ
pTis (Paget):	Paget's disease of the nipple, not associated with DCIS and/or invasive carcinoma in the underlying breast parenchyma
pT1:	Tumor ≤20 mm in greatest dimension
pT1mi:	Tumor ≤1 mm in greatest dimension
pT1a:	Tumor >1 mm but ≤5 mm in greatest dimension (round any measurement >1.0–1.9 mm to 2 mm)
pT1b:	Tumor >5 mm but ≤10 mm in greatest dimension
pT1c:	Tumor >10 mm but ≤20 mm in greatest dimension
pT2:	Tumor >20 mm but ≤50 mm in greatest dimension
pT3:	Tumor >50 mm in greatest dimension
pT4:	Tumor of any size with direct extension to the chest wall and/or to the skin (ulceration or skin nodules)
pT4a:	Extension to the chest wall; invasion or adherence to pectoralis muscle in the absence of invasion of chest wall structures does not qualify as T4
pT4b:	Ulceration and/or ipsilateral macroscopic satellite nodules and/or edema (including peau d'orange) of the skin that does not meet the criteria for inflammatory carcinoma
pT4c:	Both T4a and T4b are present
pT4d:	Inflammatory carcinoma

Lymph node categories are subdivided as the follows:

Category (pN)

pNX:	Regional lymph nodes cannot be assessed (e.g., not removed for pathological study or previously removed)
pN0:	No regional lymph node metastasis identified or ITCs only
pN0 (i+):	ITCs only (malignant cell clusters no larger than 0.2 mm) in regional lymph node(s)

pN0 (mol+):	Positive molecular findings by reverse transcriptase polymerase chain reaction (RT-PCR); no ITCs detected
pN1mi:	Micrometastases (approximately 200 cells, larger than 0.2 mm, but none larger than 2.0 mm)
pN1a:	Metastases in 1 to 3 axillary lymph nodes, at least 1 metastasis larger than 2.0 mm
pN1b:	Metastases in ipsilateral internal mammary sentinel nodes, excluding ITCs
pN1c:	pN1a and pN1b combined
pN2a:	Metastases in 4 to 9 axillary lymph nodes (at least 1 tumor deposit larger than 2.0 mm)
pN2b:	Metastases in clinically detected internal mammary lymph nodes with or without microscopic confirmation; with pathologically negative axillary nodes
pN3a:	Metastases in 10 or more axillary lymph nodes (at least 1 tumor deposit larger than 2.0 mm) or metastases to the infraclavicular (Level III axillary lymph) nodes
pN3b:	pN1a or pN2a in the presence of cN2b (positive internal mammary nodes by imaging); or pN2a in the presence of pN1b
pN3c:	Metastases in ipsilateral supraclavicular lymph nodes

Distant Metastasis (pM) stage is required only if confirmed pathologically:

pM1:	Histologically proven metastases larger than 0.2 mm Specify site, if known:_____

Residual tumor and surgical margins: (for invasive carcinoma and DCIS). *The R categories for the primary tumor site are:*
- R0 No residual tumor
- R1 Microscopic residual tumor
- R2 Macroscopic residual tumor
- RX Presence of residual tumor cannot be assessed

The margin status may be recorded using the following categories:
- Negative margins (tumor not present at surgical margin)

- Microscopic positive margin (tumor not identified grossly at the margin, but present microscopically at the margin)
- Macroscopic positive margin (tumor identified grossly at the margin)
- Margin not assessed

The R category is not incorporated into TNM staging but the status of the margins is often recorded in the medical record and cancer registry.

What is inflammatory breast cancer?

Inflammatory breast cancer has the worst prognosis of all breast cancers. Fortunately, it is rare and accounts for only 1–5% of all breast cancers in the US, mostly due to preventive care. For inflammatory breast cancer, the median survival is 2.9 years, and five-year survival rate is <45%. Inflammatory breast cancers start as Stage III (T4d,Nx,M0) and if the cancer has spread outside the breast to distant site, it is Stage IV. Pathological finding is tumor microemboli in the superficial dermal lymphatics which causes peau d'orange, a lymphedema and thickening of skin. T4d, inflammatory carcinoma requires both clinical presentation of inflammatory cancer changes and superficial dermal lymphatic microemboli of tumor cells pathologically.

Clinical manifestation of inflammatory breast cancer includes diffuse erythema, edema, peau d'orange involving at least a third or more of the skin overlying the breast and is classified as cT4d. The patients with neglected locally advanced breast cancer that may be fungated or ulcerated skin do not qualify as inflammatory breast cancer.

If clinically suspicious symptoms such as edema and peau d'orange in the absence of pathologic changes, it is staged as T4b. The presence of the dermal lymphatic tumor microemboli without the clinical findings of inflammatory carcinoma is not defined as inflammatory breast cancer.

The first treatment for the inflammatory breast cancer is chemotherapy prior to surgery, in hopes of shrinking the tumor.

How is the clinical staging of breast cancer done?

To determine the clinical stage of the breast cancer, the patient usually will see an oncologic breast surgeon. From the initial consultation, the patient is expected to have a physical examination, further imaging analysis, and blood testing for staging purposes. For further imaging analysis, the patient must make an appointment with the radiology department. For stage IV breast cancer, depending on where the metastases occur, there will be signs and symptoms. For instance, if the metastasis occurs in the brain, the patient may have memory loss, vision changes, dizziness, or specific motor problems such as falls or loss of consciousness. Depending on the specific symptoms, the oncologic breast surgeon may order different imaging.

Chapter 13:
Do men get breast cancer?

Yes. According to the *American Cancer Society*, estimates for breast cancer in men in the United States for 2021 are:

About 2,650 new cases of invasive breast cancer will be diagnosed.

About 530 men will die from breast cancer.

For men, the lifetime risk of getting breast cancer is about 1 in 833.

In comparison, breast cancer in women in the United States for 2021 are:

An estimated 281,550 new cases of invasive breast cancer are expected to be diagnosed in women in the US, along with 49,290 new cases of non-invasive (DCIS) breast cancer.

About 43,600 women are expected to die in 2021 from breast cancer. The overall death rate from breast cancer decreased by 1% per year from 2013 to 2018 and this is thought to be the result of treatment advances and earlier detection through screening.

Overall, one in eight US women (13%) will develop invasive breast cancer over the course of their lifetime.

Breast cancer is about 100 times less common among white men than among white women, and 70 times less common among Black men than Black women.

I had a 65-year-old male patient, CEO of his company, come to the ultrasound suite for an FNA biopsy. A radiologist colleague asked me to perform an FNA procedure after finding a small, approximately 1.0 cm mass in the patient's right breast. I remembered he was so ashamed and embarrassed of his condition. His discomfort and frustration were obvious to me. "I can't believe this is happening to me. I thought breast cancer is for women. I am a man and how can I have breast cancer? I am in the mammogram suite where all the people are women. I had to sit around them and wait just like one of them to get the mammogram. Then, I was brought here to the ultrasound room and now what is this you are going to do to me?"

I had to realize his humiliation was perhaps rooted from sitting among all women in a patients' waiting room, going into a locker room among mostly women to change into a gown, a woman technician performing mammograms, a female radiologist doing ultrasound test and now another female doctor performing an FNA procedure. I explained the statistics for male incidences of breast cancer, prognosis is similar stage-by-stage to women, but because male breast cancer is detected in earlier stage, their survival rate is better. Also, male breast cancers are generally smaller with a lower grade type which is better than a larger cancer of the more aggressive kind. But because many men do not realize that they can develop breast cancer, they don't seek medical attention until it reaches a later stage.

I told him I was glad that he escaped the latter scenario. I asked him about his family history of genetic mutations such as BRCA1 and BRCA2 genes, heavy alcohol consumption, liver disease, pituitary problems, radiation exposure, prostatic cancer with estrogen-related drugs and past history of mumps as an adult or undescended one or both testicles, or orchiectomy. These are the risk factors for the male breast cancers. He denied everything and was proud of the fact that he had both testicles appropriately positioned and functional, and said, "I have two grown children who have finished college." After what I explained to him, he was much more comfortable about his breast condition, knowing that he is not the only one who is undergoing such experiences and he seemed much more sympathetic to women who face losing breasts due to cancer.

What is the breast cancer risk for transgender experience?
Risk data is limited at this time. According to the Netherlands' experience *(BMJ 2019;365:l1652, 2019)*, the study showed the overall incidence of breast cancer for trans women and trans men combined was 43 per 100,000. For transgender people who experience an incongruence between the sex assigned at birth and expressed gender, breast cancer risk has been related to endocrine treatment.

In trans women (male sex assigned at birth, female gender identity), who received sex steroids consisting of antiandrogen and estrogen had higher risk (46-fold) in breast cancer than cisgender (male sex assigned at birth, male gender identity). The most common breast cancer is invasive ductal carcinoma, resembling a more female pattern.

In trans men (female sex assigned at birth, male gender identity), who received testosterone treatment had lower than expected breast cancer risk than cisgender (female sex assigned at birth and female gender identity).

I saw one trans patient who received a high dose of estrogen therapy resulting in malignant phyllodes tumor with liposarcomatous features unilaterally weighing 1,500 grams (1.5 kg) within less than one year.

Chapter 14:
To err is human

The Institute of Medicine (IOM) released a report in November 1999, *To Err is Human: Building a Safer Health System.* IOM reported that the "Health care professionals have customarily viewed errors as a sign of an individual's incompetence or recklessness. As a result, rather than learning from such events and using information to improve safety and prevent new events, health care professionals have had difficulty admitting or even discussing adverse events or *near misses,* often because they fear professional censure, administrative blame, lawsuits, or personal feelings of shame." Acknowledging this, the report put forth a four-part plan that applies to all who are, or will be, at the front lines of patient care: clinical administrators; regulating, accrediting, and licensing groups; boards of directors; industry; and government agencies. It also suggested actions that patients and their families could take to improve safety.

An article from *The New York Times* mentions the benefit of having a second opinion. *Doubt About Pathology Opinions for Early Breast Cancer* in July 2010 talks about the very issue that pathology errors can put women at risk for unnecessary and disfiguring surgeries. It further discusses potential harmful radiation treatments and horrible psychological effects resulting from errors. The article specifically describes a 30-year-old registered nurse diagnosed with a precancerous ductal carcinoma in-situ (DCIS) by a small community hospital pathologist. To put fuel onto the fire, a well-known academic pathologist during an interview said there are studies showing that diagnosing borderline breast lesions occasionally comes down to a flip of a coin.

To stress this very point, *The Journal of the American Medical Association (JAMA)* published an article in May 2015 basically comparing community hospital setting pathologists to three expert breast pathologists who wrote textbooks in the field of breast pathology. The good news was that when it comes to invasive breast cancer diagnosis, there was 96% concordance between community and academic pathologists. The bad news was a difference in opinion among a substantial percentage (16% in DCIS and 52% in atypia) between community and academic pathologists. The *JAMA* article did not emphasize the fact that the overall agreement between the three experts was 75%, and agreement among community pathologists was 75.3%. Also, the article did not stress the impractical and flawed methodology published in the article. For example, the three experts each sent one slide from 60 to 115 cases to community pathologists without any clinical information. Excluded was information on mammographic findings, whether the core biopsy was done for calcifications, mass lesion, architectural distortion, and radiologist's BI-RADS score which is the likelihood of malignant lesion from the radiologist's impression. Most importantly, the study did not include the outcome from the patient population clinically. In another words, the gold standard end point is unknown; if the lesion was called DCIS or atypia, did the excisional biopsy have DCIS or atypia? The goal of the study was to find out how the community pathologists stacked up against the academic breast expert pathologists. Remarkably, a key finding cited by the study was that the experts came to a consensus diagnosis between themselves (merely 3 pathologists), while the community pathologists did not have consensus. (Meaning they did not arrive at the same conclusion as these 3 academic pathologists).

In a real practice setting, whether one is in community practice or an expert pathologist in an academic institution, pathologists perform IHC stains and deeper recut sections to study the borderline lesions, and we share slides among colleagues to have a consensus diagnosis. Also, we discuss imaging findings with radiologists to make sure what we see in the slides match with radiological findings. In my previous academic institution, pathologists and radiologists meet every Friday to compare imaging and pathologic findings from all patients who underwent core needle biopsy that week.

The articles from *JAMA* and *The New York Times* represent a cross section of pathology practice in a worst light. In fact, other disciplines may have a higher percentage of disagreement in their opinions; I know that radiologists argue which lesions need to get biopsied and which lesions only need a follow-up in interval mammogram. Also, there are numerous differing opinions in surgical care, and varying opinions between oncologists which drug(s) to treat a patient in remarkably similar scenarios. I suspect the differences of opinion within other specialties will have a higher discordant rate than pathology. Pathologists are often in the spotlight among doctors in a hospital because we provide the final diagnosis. If the pathologist is wrong, all physicians downstream including surgeons, oncologists, and radiology-oncologists will go down a wrong path and provide the wrong care for a patient.

My impression regarding pathology errors is that everyone is fallible, whether a pathologist is from a community setting or an academic setting. Even experts can make mistakes in diagnosis. However, it is better to review the same slides by a second pathologist, especially if the patient is receiving further management such as surgery from a different institution. The best time to have a second opinion is after core needle biopsy and not after excision, which is a definitive surgery that may disfigure the breast.

One of my professors said, "If you are not making mistakes, you are not practicing." In fact, physicians "practice" medicine to become an expert in their fields every day through experiences and empirical learning. In medical practice, there is no doctrine or only one correct way, but striving to face the greatest challenges to learn, use, share and update better information, guidelines, and recommendations about how to help and to prevent harm to patients, establishing evidence-based learning.

Within the pathology laboratory is a pathologist, a human doctor, who makes the diagnosis based largely on a patient's tissue samples. We know that even machines need daily calibration to make sure they run without an error, and human doctors need constant vigilance to avoid mistakes in making diagnoses which will affect patients' lives. I tell my pathology residents we are expected to hit the baseball homerun every time, whether the pitch is a strike or ball, curveball, or fastball. I know no baseball player who can possibly produce a homerun every single time in human history and yet this is what is expected from pathologists. We must make absolutely no mistakes in making diagnoses. I also know no pathologist who never made a mistake. The only way a pathologist can avoid making mistakes is not to practice at all.

For pathologists, and other physicians, we should understand that we are merely humans, and occasional errors are inevitable. When we find out or discover the mistake, we should admit it from the very beginning and not hide it. By hiding the mistake, the harm to a patient usually snowballs, becoming larger and larger with detrimental effects to both the patient and doctor. A road to recovery is much easier if the doctor informs the patient immediately of what just happened.

One of my colleagues, recently hired after completing his fellowship training, "read out" a patient's breast core needle biopsy as "invasive ductal carcinoma, grade 1," but in reality, the patient only had a benign condition named "sclerosing adenosis" which can mimic invasive carcinoma. The pathologist ordered no immunohistochemical stains to confirm the nature of invasive carcinoma. The patient underwent a mastectomy rather than a breast-conserving lumpectomy because the patient did not want to deal with possible positive margin and radiation therapy which takes multiple trips to a medical center.

On the mastectomy specimen, there was no residual carcinoma from the prior biopsy site, but sclerosing adenosis was found adjacent to the microclip placed after the core biopsy site by the radiologist. The original slide from the core biopsy sample was re-reviewed and immunohistochemical stains performed to confirm a benign lesion from the core biopsy sample, as well as the mastectomy sample. The pathologist called the surgeon and admitted his mistake. The surgeon was incredibly frustrated with this but immediately called the patient with this news.

The patient came to see the surgeon a few days later for a routine follow-up to remove sutures and told the surgeon, "Well, at least there is no cancer in my breast! I don't need to have a breast when I am almost 70 years old." The patient did not press charges against the pathologist. It is a sobering story for pathologists that we should never take our job lightly.

On the contrary, some patients jump on any opportunity either not to pay the pathology bills and/or sue the pathologist and the hospital for monetary gain if they suspect any possible error.

I have seen a patient who had a small pea-sized nipple adenoma, a benign growth underneath the nipple which required removal with clear margin. On a skin punch biopsy of the nipple, the main mass underneath the nipple was not sampled – only the superficial skin with a clinical history of "scaling lesion." The pathologist had seen few atypical cells in the skin epidermis and signed out in the report stating, "We cannot entirely rule out Paget's disease." A wider excision was performed by a surgeon who needed to remove the entire pea-sized tumor and the skin tissue. On the excision, there was no diagnostic residual Paget's disease. Because the procedure was designated as a "mastectomy" due to the inclusion of the nipple and a portion of the areolar complex around the nipple, the patient sued the pathologist.

She also demanded plastic surgery to recreate her nipple to have better cosmetic results and breast augmentation by silicone implants, all for free of charge. With a diagnosis of Paget's disease in the nipple skin, there is almost 100% chance of having at least DCIS if not invasive breast carcinoma. The surgeon could have done mastectomy. But the surgeon did not take out her breast tissue, just the tissue under the nipple and the entire specimen measured 1.0 cm.

I have seen extremely gracious patients and nasty patients in my practice. Either way, as a pathologist, I do my best to serve the patients under the Hippocratic oath, "Do no harm."

Chapter 15:
How to be an effective clinician who works with pathologists

Over the past 25 years of pathology practice, I notice things change. Fewer and fewer surgical residents are coming through pathology rotations as a part of their training. This is unfortunate because surgeons are intimate partners with pathologists whether they like it or not.

It is critical to patient care that surgeons understand how a pathologist conducts their business after tissue is surgically removed. Pathologists and surgeons should not work in their vacuum. I often receive patients' tissue without any clinical history, nor why the clinician biopsied the tissue. It feels like certain clinicians are saying, "Guess what I am thinking?" I understand that clinicians are very busy with their practice but taking time to fill out the surgical pathology requisition form appropriately with the best contact phone number or email is always appreciated. It is critical for accurate pathology diagnosis leading to best patient care to know the patient's history: Where is the lesion from? What is the size of the lesion? What is the complete history of the patient especially the previous cancer history, and what are the specific questions from the clinician?

I performed an FNA biopsy of the thyroid on a patient who had a 3.5 cm mass. The FNA specimen was unusually bloody even though I used a tiny needle. After staining, the cells from the patient had a malignancy but did not "fit" any of the primary thyroid cancers. After much pondering, I decided to rule out a metastatic renal cell carcinoma (kidney cancer) and ordered appropriate IHC stains to confirm. It turns out that the patient had a prior renal cell carcinoma 10 years prior and had a surgery in another institution which I discovered only after calling the clinician. This case would have been so much easier if I had known this history and not wasted resources for additional IHC stains to prove that it was not a primary thyroid carcinoma.

In my opinion, the best clinicians and surgeons often come to the pathologist's office and review slides under the microscope with the pathologist, and/or include the interesting and unusual cases in tumor boards. Inevitably, communication is enhanced during this time, especially if the case is unusual and leads to better patient care.

The primary concern in real estate is "location, location and location," but in medicine, the best care for patients is "communicate, communicate and communicate." Communication is challenging from the clinician's point of view. They are normally required to see patients within a 15–20 minute window, have good bedside manners, document all their findings with future management plans in their electronic medical record system, and perform thorough physical examinations. Managed Care is asking doctors to be more efficient which means restraining use of our time to help patients—including pathologists. We are often required to see more slides within a given time, and to perform fewer IHC or ancillary tests to arrive at a diagnosis.

Communication with pathologists is one way to solve unnecessary ancillary testing costs and deliver the best care for our patients. Most pathologists appreciate clinical colleagues' provision of our patients' information and medical history.

IV. The next steps for a patient

Chapter 16:
What to do when you face a cancer diagnosis?

Cancer is the second or third most common cause of death depending on different age groups. Many of us go through a tough time and a long journey to deal with a cancer diagnosis. The first phase is shock. The next phase is asking why and at times seeking answers from God if a patient is religious. The next phase is anger and finally an acceptance stage. When one begins to lose control, or is in fear and doubt, having a quiet moment to gather your thoughts and know what to expect in the medical world will better help you face the reality. First, complete all the prescribed medical procedures. If it is breast cancer, you likely will already have a diagnosis of cancer by the core needle biopsy result. The next phase is to see a breast surgeon and get the initial consultation. This step is to figure out if you are eligible for a surgical procedure.

Knowledge is power. Informed patients are better at dealing with their cancer diagnosis. Be ready to educate yourself with breast cancer. The best educational resources are from professional, trusted sources (most likely not social media). Start with your doctor's educational materials and resources, or other information they may provide.

Once you have a diagnosis of breast cancer, the world may appear to go upside down and you may face loss of control in your life. There are a few specific things you can do to gain some control over your life. It will be a journey and not an event and therefore, keep a diary for this journey.

These are my suggestions that may help you to organize:
- Get a notebook/three ring binder to keep a daily diary for you to use, starting from the date you receive a diagnosis of cancer.
- Get a calendar with this notebook.

- Keep track of all appointments with your surgeon, radiologist-oncologist, oncologist etc.
- Keep a "to-do-list" every day and check off each item.
- Ask family, friends, and perhaps those who attend synagogue, temple, monastery or church to help you. Do not hesitate to seek help especially if you are to receive chemotherapy.
- Prayers
- Meals
- House cleaning
- Driving arrangements
- Family obligations such as your children's needs

For the earlier stages of the breast cancer, surgery is usually the first option of treatment. After the surgical excision, other treatments may include radiation and chemotherapy. You may or may not need radiation and/or chemotherapy.

After staging analysis, you will need to see your oncology surgeon again to discuss whether surgical treatment is a plan for you. Necessary questions usually consist of **what, when, where, how,** and **why**. Because it is overwhelming to understand and follow the conversations with medical professionals, it is a good idea to bring someone else who can listen during the consultation time and record the process. Make sure you tell the surgeon and get their approval for recording the conversation before you start recording. Some may not like the idea of recording the medical consultation. Take your time to get all the answers to your questions. This is your time with the doctors and the more you understand what needs to be done, the better you will gain some control over your health.

During the appointment with your surgeon, the following questions will most likely prove helpful for you:
1. How large is the tumor?
2. Did it appear to spread to the axillary lymph nodes?
3. Did the tumor spread to chest wall or skin?
4. Did the tumor spread outside of the breast and axillary lymph node?
5. What is the grade of the tumor?

6. What are the prognostic biomarkers of the tumor? ER, PR, Her-2/*neu* status and Ki-67?
7. Was there lymphovascular invasion from the core needle biopsy?
8. Is there a benefit to do neoadjuvant chemotherapy (chemotherapy before the surgery)?
9. What are my options for surgery? Lumpectomy or mastectomy?
10. Is the sentinel lymph node necessary?
11. Is the axillary lymph node dissection necessary?
12. When is the surgery? How soon can it be done?
13. What are the cosmetic options after or during surgery?
14. Where will be the incisional site?
15. How long is the surgery and what will be expected after the surgery?
16. Is there possibility of blood transfusion during surgery? What is my blood type and any unusual or expected transfusion reactions?
17. What will be limiting factors after the surgery? Arm range of motion, swelling, pain etc.
18. What and how long to take pain medications? What are other options for pain medication when trying to avoid narcotics?
19. When can I go back to work? When can I resume my normal activities as usual after surgery?
20. How many days after surgery must I wait before taking a shower?
21. What are the complications or signs of problems, and who do I call if I experience any of these complications?
22. What happens after the surgery? Are there follow-up appointments, with whom and when?
23. Will I need to be hospitalized after the surgery, and if so, how long?
24. Are there any written instructions or educational materials for me to read?
25. Is there a phone number and person I can call to ask questions?

Consider taking care of these things prior to surgery or other procedures:

- *Health Insurance Portability and Accountability Act (HIPAA) form* signed by the patient if you want anyone from your family or your friends to be involved with your medical care. You must sign this form with their names. Doctors and nurses are not allowed to discuss anything over the phone or in person about the patient to family members or friends, even if you or they are health care providers, for privacy and safety to protect the patient. Only you as the patient can specifically ask certain persons to be involved in your medical care. HIPAA forms can be obtained in the hospital or clinic and only the patient can sign, which then allows your medical institution or health care personnel to share your medical information.

- *Do Not Resuscitate (DNR) form*—discuss with your doctor and bring any legal form you may already have filled out. In case you are not able to make appropriate judgment for yourself, it is important to decide specifically which of your next kin, or who you choose to give "power of attorney" that can make the best decisions for your best interest. Death is a possibility anytime you go through a major or even minor surgery, and prior to any surgery you will sign a consent form with a long list of possible side effects of surgery including death.

24 hours before, during and after surgery:

- You will be asked not to eat or drink 24 hours before the surgery.
- Arrive at the hospital or clinic at least two hours before the surgery is scheduled to check in.
- It is best to schedule the first surgery in the morning if you can.
- The surgery schedule often gets delayed, so do not be alarmed when you go to surgery much later than your expected time, especially if yours is not the first surgery of the day, or if your surgeon has another surgery scheduled before yours.
- During the recovery after surgery, the surgeon will come out to meet the family members and/or friends. There may be specific instructions and you will need to have someone with you to listen and take notes.

- After surgery, you will be on pain medication(s) and probably not alert and able to drive. However, you may be discharged from the hospital or clinic shortly after surgery and therefore, you will need a family member or friend to drive you home.
- If you need to be hospitalized, it would be best to have a family member to remain with you, be at your bedside, and be present when the doctors are doing their rounds (usually quite early in the morning). Ask nurses when your doctor does "rounding." Medical professionals are there to help you and their patients, but in my experience "the squeaky wheel" gets their attention first.

Questions to ask doctors during your discharge:
1. Should I continue all my medications as before? (Bring the list of all your medications)
2. What dosage? Example, hypertension medication.
3. When can I take a shower? When can I go to the pool (if you are a swimmer)?
4. If I get constipation after morphine or other narcotic pain medication, what can I take to make my stool softer?
5. What should I expect for complications such as signs of bleeding, infection, obstruction, or other signs to look for?
6. When are the follow-up appointments and which doctors will I see?
7. Do I need home nursing care for drainage, and changing the gauze for the wound?

After the surgery, you will most likely meet with your breast surgeon in about one week to 10 days after the surgical procedure. This is because the pathology report will be out, which may take some time.

Questions to ask to your surgeon about your pathology report:
1. How large is the tumor? The tumor size may be different from the clinical or imaging size because the pathologist will look at the tumor via a microscope, the most accurate sizing method.
2. Was there more than one site of tumor (multifocal tumors)?
3. Lymph node metastasis? How many lymph nodes did the pathologist find?
4. What is the size of metastasis in the lymph node?

5. If there is metastasis to lymph node, were the tumor cells found outside the lymph node (extranodal extension)? Extranodal extension has poor prognosis.
6. Was the surgical margin clear?
7. What grade is it? Grade 1, 2 or 3?
8. Is there lymphovascular invasion (LVI)?
9. What is the stage of the tumor?
10. What are the biomarkers (ER, PR and Her-2/*neu*) from the excision and are they different from the core needle biopsy sample?
11. What is the prognosis?
12. Do I need to have chemotherapy? What kind of chemotherapy, how long? What are the side effects of each chemotherapy regimen?
13. Do I need to have radiation therapy?
14. Do I need hormonal therapy and for how long?
15. How long might I live if I do not receive chemotherapy or radiation therapy? If the surgeon is vague or does not provide an answer, you can ask, *"What does the medical literature suggest about life expectancy?"*
16. What is my expected schedule for surveillance?
17. Is there a support group for me and for my family members?
18. If I want a second opinion for treatment options or second opinion for pathology review, what are the steps?
19. Who do you think I should see for the second opinions, and why?

Ask for the paper printouts of all the medical documents including pathology reports, radiology reports and surgical dictations. Certain hospitals may not provide you with all these reports because of their policies. Your surgeon may not answer all these questions, but your oncologist and radiation oncologist doctors can answer most if not all these questions.

As I outlined before, it is important to organize your life so that you will have some control over your life. Think through the finances, get "your house in order" including your will, and get them done when possible. There are multiple tasks to think through and do. Currently, breast cancer patients often survive for many years, some even beyond 10 years. But this is the opportunity to at least think about your loved ones, your will, beneficiaries, your own funeral arrangements, and donations.

Getting back to a healthy life includes a spiritual component I recommend the patient to consider. Encouragement and positive human contacts from friends and family members are significant in the pathway to recovery, including communications with God if religion is part of one's life. One sure thing in life is death. Everyone will die at some point and death is inevitable. However, we do not need to live in fear of death. We need to live life during the time we have breath. Everyone goes through their healing process differently.

Some patients become quiet and reserved; this may be related to cultural upbringing. Some Japanese patients are often shocked to find out that in the US, cancer patients have a shared chemotherapy infusion room, allowing patients to see and talk to other patients for several hours as they undergo infusion treatments. American patients may not understand why a common space for chemotherapy infusion would not be desired. Japanese patients stricken with cancer are sometimes secretive and suffer their pain alone, quietly. I cannot comment on how best to resolve getting through the phases of emotional and spiritual suffering during times of chemotherapy and radiation therapy, but for me, documenting the experiences in a diary and daily talks/prayers with God may be the most comforting tasks.

I found this *Balance Sheet of Life* which may have originated from the Persian poet, Rumi. A quotation by Rumi reads, "The WOUND is the place where LIGHT enters." **Rumi's balance sheet of life:**

The most destructive habit	*Worry*
The greatest joy	*Giving*
The greatest loss	*Loss of self-respect*
The ugliest personality trait	*Selfishness*
The most satisfying work	*Helping others*
The greatest "shot in the arm"	*Encouragement*
The greatest problem to overcome	*Fear*
The most effective sleeping pill	*Peace of mind*
The most crippling failure disease	*Excuses*
The most powerful force in life	*Love*
The most dangerous act	*A gossip*
The world's most incredible computer	*The brain*
The worst thing to be without	*Hope*
The deadliest weapon	*The tongue*
The most power-filled words	*I can*
The greatest asset	*Faith*
The most worthless emotion	*Self-pity*
The most beautiful attire	*Smile*
The most prized possessions	*Integrity*
The most powerful channel of communication	*Prayer*
The most contagious spirit	*Enthusiasm*

Chapter 17:
Is the second opinion necessary?

Sometimes a patient will ask for a second opinion from a pathology department. It can be intradepartmental or interdepartmentally. Intradepartmental second opinion is asking a different pathologist to review the slide within the same institution. Interdepartmental is seeking the second opinion from an entirely different institution within the same state or different states.

One of my patients asked me for a second opinion in the radiology suite during an FNA procedure, even before receiving the specimen. I asked the patient, "How do you know you want a second opinion when you haven't even received the first opinion?" Many patients have a preconceived notion that the second opinion is more correct than the first opinion for reasons unknown to me, perhaps a mistrust in medical system. Other patients never doubt doctors and trust their doctor no matter what is being said.

For the patients, it is difficult to know when and when not to have the second opinion. If one wants to have a second opinion from a pathologist, the best time for a patient to request a second opinion is after the core needle biopsy. An accurate reading of the core needle biopsy is important to confirm benign or malignancy before undergoing any further surgery or neoadjuvant chemotherapy based on a potentially false positive misdiagnosis for cancer. Conversely, to prevent a false negative misdiagnosis, a benign diagnosis can be confirmed by a second pathologist's opinion and avoid a delay in diagnosis. Majority of the time, the second pathologist agrees with the first pathologist's diagnosis. However, there are rare occasions of a discordance in diagnosis between the two pathologists, which can be dramatic, such as benign to malignant or malignant to benign lesion. This circumstance occurs not only in breast pathology but many other organ systems as well. In such cases, the pathologist needs to contact the treating doctors to inform the major discordant diagnosis, and a courtesy call to the original pathologist.

There are two distinct types of discordances: major and minor. A major discordant case is when the diagnosis would end up in a significantly different treatment and management such as benign to malignant diagnosis. A minor discordant case, for instance, is when the grade of the malignant tumor is changed from grade 1 to 2 and resulting in no differences in the management. The minor discordant cases are more common, and no phone calls are needed to both the treating doctors and the original pathologist.

It is not unusual that a patient undergoes a core needle biopsy at one institution, and the excisional biopsy surgery at another institution. In this scenario, I would recommend that all outside pathology slides be reviewed at the final institution where the patient is planning to have surgery, radiation and/or chemotherapy to prevent both overtreatment and undertreatment. Detecting the latter case of undertreatment can be more difficult. For example, if the original pathologist diagnoses a benign lesion in the breast of a particular patient in a small biopsy sample, the patient will most likely trust the diagnosis and simply follow up with their next annual mammogram unless the mass continues to grow and becomes symptomatic. However, preventing overtreatment of the case can be avoided by requiring a review of the outside slides. This policy is healthy whenever a patient is referred to a doctor or treatment at an institution other than the one where the primary diagnosis was rendered, but not all hospitals mandate this policy.

The clinician, whether it is a surgeon, radiation oncologist or oncologist should ask the patient to obtain the original pathology slides. These pathology slides were generated for the final diagnosis, and hence they are the most important aspect of the patient's downstream management. This process may be complicated and confusing for the patient who may not know the medical policies or the facility well enough to contact the pathology department or who to talk to, especially in time of distress with a bad diagnosis such as "cancer."

To further complicate matters, the patient will be asked to sign a HIPAA form, go to the original facility, and obtain the glass slides that are accompanied by detailed instructions on how to care for the slides. Glass slides are fragile and easily broken and need to be handled with caution. In addition, the stained glass slides may fade under direct sunlight and should be covered and placed in a cool dark area, or at least within normal room temperature. The patient can also ask the original pathology department to send the slides to the other institution, which is the most common and preferred way.

The original slides belong to the pathology department and are retained partly because they may become critical in medical-legal situations. Most departments make copies of the slides; we call these "recut" slides for second opinions. Recut slides are nearly identical to the original slides, but not all recut slides show the exact same features as the original slides. As a rare example, a recut slide might show small metastatic carcinoma in a lymph node when the original slide did not, or vice versa. Or, the original slide might show tumor at the inked margin, while the recut slide could show no ink, or tumor not actually touching at the inked margin. If a recut slide shows more disease not seen from the original slide, the pathologist who is releasing the recut slide will make an amendment/corrected diagnosis. If the original slide only shows the lesional tissue, then, the original slide will be released to the second institution. When a recut is made, the patient must pay additional fees, usually $5 to $10 per slide depending on the hospital policy. The costs can add up to a significant amount if the slides are from an excisional biopsy such as partial mastectomy, or mastectomy cases with lymph nodes dissection. For this reason, the original pathologist may send only the key slides for diagnostic confirmation.

Pathologists often deal with difficult cases by using multiple methods of appropriately handling of each case. We often consult with each other and show cases with one another, sometimes many pathologists. We can also perform additional ancillary tests called Immunohistochemical (IHC) stains. IHC stains may help to delineate many difficult cases. Consultation with an outside institution is also an option for the pathologist who personally sends a case for consultation. Pathologists who are known experts in breast pathology are in many major academic university hospitals and in certain private practice settings.

Institutions prefer not to release their original IHC slides because it then becomes more difficult to make recuts, costly to reproduce, and it risks the original slides becoming lost. The pathologist from the outside consulting institution may just have to rely on the original pathologist's interpretations of the IHC stain results. The second pathologist can also request the original pathologist to send the tissue block out to repeat or add additional IHC stains as needed to provide an accurate diagnosis. Providing an accurate diagnosis is the ultimate goal for all pathologists; and hence, the original facility will send the tissue block or multiple unstained slides with proper documentation and tracing. Once the second pathologist receives the block, the responsibility of damage or loss is shifted to the second institution. Careful records of slides and tissue block tracing is particularly important in all pathology departments.

Generally, a patient finds out who their pathologist is by two scenarios. First, hospital bills include pathology expenses. Patients may call hospital billing departments and ask, "Why am I paying for pathology?" The second scenario is when a surgeon or radiologist points to a pathologist who "made a mistake" in their diagnosis. This rarely occurs, but it happens. Pathologists are humans and all humans are prone to make mistakes. We all know this and yet when doctors make mistakes, somehow it is more unforgivable and unforgettable because after all, there is a patient who will be suffering at the end. So, a pathologist in any part of a conversation with patient care is often not seen in a good light. Even if the baseball batting average for a pathologist is 99 out of 100, just one strikeout will be magnified a thousand times because there is a patient at the receiving end who experienced considerable damage. Pathologists do not intend to make any mistake.

I experienced a few patients who refused to allow a pathology report to be sent along with their slides because of fear that the second opinion would be biased toward the original diagnostic opinion. The pathology report must accompany the slides because the pathology report provides essential information such as a description of gross, clinical information, number of slides submitted to match the actual number of glass slides, location(s), date of procedure, the details of the original pathologist's impression along with IHC stain results and detailed billing information. Since a pathologist does not see the patient's face to identify the correct patient, it is critically important that we see the same slides as reported in the original pathology report. What a patient may not realize is that the second opinion pathologist is not necessarily "biased" by the first pathologist's diagnosis. Most diagnoses are straightforward and not difficult. For all these reasons, our institution will not accept outside slides without the pathology report and the billing information. Often, the second opinion facility will return the slides within one to two months to the original facility by overnight or two-day delivery with a tracking number for verification. In rare situations the slides are returned directly to the patient, but only by the patient's request.

As an expert breast pathologist in a major academic setting, I received hundreds and perhaps thousands of second opinion slides from patients and their clinicians. One case stands out in my personal experiences.

The patient had a 2.0 cm mass lesion detected by both mammogram and ultrasound imaging and underwent a core needle biopsy. The original pathologist signed out the case as a breast carcinoma, triple negative type (ER, PR and Her-2/neu negative) but noticed that the glands were rather well formed, low nuclear grade and low mitotic figures with a modified Bloom and Richardson score of 4 out of 9, grade 1 tumor. (It is very unusual for a grade 1 breast cancer to have triple negativity. Nearly all grade 1 tumors are strongly positive for ER and PR, and negative for Her-2/neu). The patient underwent a lumpectomy and a sentinel lymph node biopsy, and the same pathologist signed out her case as a breast carcinoma, grade 1, 2.0 cm in size, with one of the six margins positive for carcinoma. The sentinel lymph node was negative for metastatic carcinoma. Again, the repeated prognostic breast biomarkers done on the lumpectomy specimen were similar as the core needle sample, triple negative.

Because of the positive margin, the patient underwent a complete mastectomy which was signed out as a small residual breast cancer and clear margin. Subsequently, the patient received a triple negative regimen chemotherapy which is the standard practice for the triple negative breast cancer, for they are known to have a poor prognosis. Upon completion of the 6 cycles of chemotherapy, the patient decided to come to our institution for a prophylactic contralateral mastectomy because she was scared to have any breast tissue left behind.

As part of our hospital policy, I reviewed all the patient's previous samples. The patient had a diagnosis of adenomyoepithelioma, which is a benign lesion and commonly triple negative. It was evident in her core biopsy, lumpectomy, and a residual lesion from the mastectomy. This patient did not require a sentinel lymph node biopsy, complete mastectomy, nor the chemotherapy. Adenomyoepithelioma is a rare lesion in the breast, often presents as a mass lesion and the treatment should be a complete excision.

This is one of the false positive interpretation errors by an original pathologist. And hence, the best time for a second opinion is after the core needle biopsy. Second opinions sometimes are not covered by insurance but in this case, the dollar amount (usually less than $200–$300) is well spent by the patient to avoid a detrimental effect.

Chapter 18:
How does a patient find an expert pathologist for a second opinion?

There are basically three ways to get an expert pathology opinion.

1. **The patient can request a second opinion directly.** The second review of the case slides can be done by intradepartmental (within the same institution) or interdepartmental (outside the institution) methods as explained previously. In rare situations, a patient may worry about intrinsic bias if an intradepartmental second opinion is provided. But most pathologists look at each case afresh without bias, and their medical license depends on the integrity of their knowledge and honesty. Most doctors, in fact, are trained to look at the case cold, without bias or favoring their doctor colleagues because it is also in the patient's best interest.

For the interdepartmental second opinion, breast pathology experts are found online, but it will be difficult to know who is "good." The choices are among institutions such as Brigham and Women's Hospital, Johns Hopkins, and University of California Los Angeles (UCLA). There are a number of breast pathology subspecialty experts who can look at your slide(s) and generate a second opinion report. Each institution has a group of people who are subspecialized in breast pathology, with varying experiences. Depending on the schedule of the day, the slide may end up with a newly hired and inexperienced breast pathologist who happens to be on duty. However, there are often more experienced breast pathologists nearby to share (internal consultation) if the case is difficult.

To request a second opinion, the patient must sign HIPAA and medical record release forms, contact the pathology department, and request a second opinion from another institution. The patient can request the pathology department send the slide(s), or the patient can retrieve the slides and personally send them to the institution of their choice. It is important to preserve the slides in a cool temperature and not directly under the sun. The slides are glass, fragile and easy to break. Pathology departments often put the slides inside specially designed glass slide holders for protection. There may be a charge for recut slides and glass slide holders. It is best to send the slides using an overnight carrier who includes traceable technology with their shipments, such as FedEx or UPS.

2. **Pathologists can ask an expert pathologist for their opinion.** It is often called a "consultation." When the case is truly challenging, the original pathologist can send out the slides, including patient medical information such as imaging results, the preliminary pathology report along with the patient's insurance information, and direct billing information as required by the pathology department. Since pathologists know each other and know who the best and trustworthy experts in breast pathology are most appropriate for their particular case, these are likely the "true experts" in the field. Most specimens are not difficult to diagnose, but approximately 5% of the time I ask myself, "What the heck is this?" if I am stunned with a case. This situation happens more commonly with frozen section procedures during an operation but can occasionally arise in the routine sign out with permanent sections.

The first thing I then do is share the slides with pathology colleagues within my department. I may or may not get additional opinions or new advice. Regardless, my next step is to explore all possible names of the disease (we call this "differential diagnosis") by ordering immunohistochemical stains to narrow down the potential diagnosis. At the same time, I do journal searches, find a similar disease(s), and print out the publications for later reading after I finish the rest of the other cases that have piled up on my desk that day.

Once I am captured by a challenge like this, it is hard not to think about the case the entire day. I can barely wait to go back to the case and figure out what it is. I continuously tell myself, "Whatever it is, it originated from the body and organs." In fact, "Everything under the sun has been described in medicine."

Finally, I read the literature and textbooks that may help describe the disease. Next day, the eagerly awaited immunohistochemical slides come out for me to review and quench my curiosity. Nearly every time I arrive at the name of the disease by the combination of all required and acquired knowledge, and ancillary tests such as immunohistochemical stains.

At times, there are cases where I am not comfortable signing out even though I probably have the likely diagnosis. I will not sign out such a case with a patient behind my slide with just my "most likely," or my "best guess." So, I will send it out to the best expert for their consultation to verify whether my likely diagnosis is correct. My own litmus test is to ask myself, "Can I sleep tonight if I sign out the case today and let it go?" If the answer is no, then I leave the case aside to review and study until at least the next day.

In my professional career, there are many sleepless nights I am preoccupied with such cases and almost obsessed with finding the proper name of the diseases. I become competitive and irritated. I cannot be peaceful and content if I have trouble figuring things out. Actually, I am in agony. The patients will never know how much their pathologist may have suffered and worked behind the scenes to provide the best name for the disease. Surgeons and patients might ask, "What's taking so long?" Obtaining an anatomic pathology report from the pathologist is different from some machine printing out the results from a lab blood test. There is a person, a medical doctor, who is looking, contemplating, and studying to provide the disease names. When the surgeon says, "We will send your tissue to the lab and will know what it is in three or four days," it means the tissue is being sent to a pathologist, not a lab; a person who is competent and sometimes fallible.

Not everything the pathologist says is always correct, for at times no human being is perfect. Note that it is the expert's opinion or pathologist's opinion on the final diagnosis; the best fitted name of the disease based on their medical knowledge and experiences. And not all expert opinions are more valid or correct than the original pathologist's opinion. Sometimes, the original pathologist may know better about clinical and imaging findings and know more about the patient's signs and symptoms than the expert pathologist, which may help to derive the correct diagnosis.

The best pathologists in my opinion understand their limits; when they do not know and when to seek help from others.

3. **Lawyers can request an expert pathology opinion.** This typically occurs when a patient sues the hospital, clinicians, or the pathologist. All medical records are stored in secured areas. This includes pathology reports, original slides, and tissue blocks. The original slides go to pathology experts for medical malpractice review. These slides are always original slides, not the recuts. These pathologists are not necessarily "true experts" in the field of breast pathology. Almost any pathologist can review lawsuit cases, and the monetary benefit attracts a variety of pathologists. Lawyers in the medical malpractice realm typically select "expert" pathologists who are currently practicing medicine (usually not retired pathologists) and have some level of name recognition, at least in their own community. Medical lawsuits are a complicated matter and there is no justice for either side. The only party to benefit from medical malpractice lawsuits are the attorneys. The patients and the doctors both lose.

Breast is the second most common field of medical malpractice lawsuit in the field of pathology. Cases of melanoma are the most litigated among all the fields of pathology. From the patient's side, misdiagnosis or overdiagnosis may delay the proper treatment or cause overtreatment, respectively, and both situations cause emotional suffering. From the doctor's point of view, the pathologists do their best in the given situations and do not mean to cause the harm. I have seen severely egregious lawsuits experienced by colleagues during my practice. Fortunately, these cases were not related to me, only observed, and frequently the patients sought large monetary gains for unusual matters.

One patient sued a surgeon for not providing the complete name of the surgical procedure on the patient consent form, naming it "Mastopexy" in addition to "Mastoplasty." Mastopexy is the name of a procedure for raising and reshaping the breasts to give them a firmer, rounder look for better cosmesis. Mastoplasty is to alter or augment the breast. The patient has a modified radical mastectomy on one breast for cancer and signed for mastoplasty for both breasts, one to cut off "dog ear," which is an extra skin fold common after suturing and silicone implant. The other breast needed to have reduction mammaplasty to match the cancer side, since the patient had large pendulous breasts and wanted to have smaller breasts. The patient was very satisfied with the end results and liked her appearance much better than before the surgery but noted that she never signed the consent form to lift her breasts, and this resulted in the lawsuit.

I know a pathologist with color blindness who signed out after misinterpreting the red and green ink at the margins. Red ink was applied to the lateral edge and green ink was applied to the medial edge of the margins. Red ink, the lateral margin, was positive for DCIS and the green-inked medial margin was negative. The pathologist signed out "DCIS was present at medial margin and the lateral margin was negative." The surgeon went back for a re-excision, and he did a circumferential (all around) the previous lumpectomy cavity, not just the medial margin. The result for cosmesis was disfigurement, especially at the medial side of the chest wall and the dissatisfied patient sued the pathologist. One may wonder why a color blind person would become a pathologist, but I personally have known great pathologists with the same condition. Pathologists are excellent at the visual and pattern recognition, and the color is not necessarily the most significant component of the practice. In this case, I wonder why the surgeon was not part of the medical lawsuit and why the color blind pathologist did not ask another pathologist to confirm red and green colors.

Another lawsuit I observed was a patient suing the radiologist who missed her invasive lobular cancer a year earlier. There are two main types of breast cancers: ductal and lobular cancers. The majority of breast cancer cases are invasive ductal cancer, while lobular cancer cases are approximately 10–15%. Interestingly, lobular carcinoma does not illicit any response from the breast tissue and often does not form a mass lesion, like ductal cancer. Radiologists look at the shadow of this breast tissue response that forms a mass in their imaging studies. This tissue response is described as "desmoplastic response" as a pathologic term. Lobular carcinoma is sneaky, causing infiltration into fat and normal breast ducts without the desmoplastic response and hence, it is rather easy to miss the lesion both by radiologists and pathologists, especially in a small biopsy sample. In this case, it was only the radiologist who missed a subtle lesion from the previous year. The patient claimed that she would have a better prognosis if detected a year earlier, but now, she had a larger tumor with lymph node metastases.

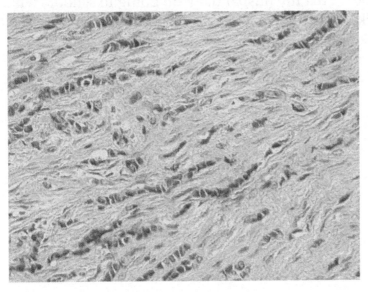

Example of invasive lobular carcinoma forming single filing and not eliciting stromal desmoplasia.

The retrospective scope is always 20/20. The expert radiologist from the plaintiff side claimed that the original radiologist obviously missed a lesion which could have been targeted for a core needle biopsy a year ago, when in fact, most radiologists would have missed the lesion without knowing the outcome for the patient. It would be reasonable to miss the lesion when the imaging is read by most radiologists in routine practices. The radiologist who was named in this lawsuit decided to settle the case and quit his practice altogether at rather young age. This case could have been won, even if the case went to the court with a jury trial because it was highly defensible for the radiologist. Doctors generally do not like conflicts and give up quickly, perhaps too easily.

It takes courage to practice medicine as a doctor. Every day brings new challenges and new findings. We, the doctors, learn new things every day, even the most experienced doctors are often astonished by the new diseases, updates and knowledge which make us humble and stay in our practice as students forever. It is truly the "practice of medicine" and never the "mastery of medicine." I tell my husband, "I am going to school" when I leave for work, even after 25 years of medical practice because I feel that I have so much to learn from medicine.

Chapter 19:
How to be an effective patient and part of the team for your health care

Knowledge is power. No one except you has more motivation and the power to change the course of your own illness. Hope dies last. Do not push the responsibilities of your health care to the hands of the doctors alone. You need to be involved in knowing everything, follow the instructions the medical team is providing, and understand why the recommendations are best for your own health care. Do not trust the doctors or the health care system entirely without question and follow through with your health issues.

For instance, a patient had a rather large mass in her breast, 3 cm, round, well defined borders detected by mammogram, and she had undergone a core needle biopsy. The pathologist signed out the lesion as a fibroadenoma, the most common benign entity in the breast. The patient was informed it was a benign lesion and hence did not worry at all, even though the lesion became larger and larger, double the size within one year. The patient waited a second year, and finally came to see her primary doctor regarding her enlarging breast mass. By now, it was stretching her skin to the point of ulceration causing pain. The mass now occupied most of her breast, larger in size than a grapefruit. When the doctor asked why she had not come for medical help earlier, the patient confidently said, "I had a diagnosis of benign fibroadenoma two years ago," which astounded the primary care doctor. The patient underwent a complete mastectomy, and the final diagnosis was a malignant phyllodes tumor.

Malignant phyllodes tumor has potential for metastasis, recurrence, and even death. An area of benign fibroadenoma can commonly be found adjacent to malignant phyllodes tumors. The core needle sample takes less than 1–5% of the entire lesion and hence, the sampling error in knowing the entire lesion is a distinct possibility. Also, in this case, the lesion may have started with a fibroadenoma and in time transformed into malignancy. Fortunately, most fibroadenoma in core needle biopsies are fibroadenoma on excision. If the mass is continuously growing, the patient needs to come back for clinical follow up and re-biopsy; or excise the entire lesion to avoid sampling error.

As the patient, you have the right to ask the medical doctors to consider your requests, whether it is regarding additional biopsy, to undergo chemotherapy or not, or undergo lumpectomy or mastectomy. A balanced discussion between you and your doctors will create the best solution for recovery. The patient has the right to know and right to choose their path in medical care. You are an integral part of your health and decision-making process. Don't be overly trusting or passive in your health care, for no one cares more about you than yourself.

On the contrary, I have seen a few patients decide not to do anything doctors recommended, explaining they believe in natural remedies to cure breast cancer. No surgery, no chemotherapy, no radiation, and no hormonal therapy — just organic food and drinks. Many of these patients returned to their medical office to get a palliative surgery to avoid necrotic, ulcerating and fungating breast cancer that smells awful. They missed the chance to cure the disease when the tumor was small enough for lumpectomy.

Another type of patient is one who trusts information stated in social media which may be misinformation or exaggerated scenarios. Medical information available in social media typically are not peer-reviewed scientific articles which most doctors and health care professions must abide. When it comes to trusting, I would trust what your doctor has to say. When in doubt, go to a reputable institution and ask them to review your case. Most reputable institutions have a multidisciplinary breast conference where all the breast specialists come together to discuss case-by-case scenarios and provide their expertise in surgery, radiology, pathology, oncology, radiation oncology, psychiatry, nursing, social work, or other fields. Patient and family cancer support groups, and cancer survivorship programs can be introduced from such institutions, and some may provide financial support if a patient is unable to pay.

For more information on breast cancer, I recommend patients visit the National Comprehensive Cancer Network website.
https://www.nccn.org/guidelines/patients

Author's final thoughts

Science is not anti-religion or anti-God. I believe God is with science and every discovery in medicine is a blessing from God to treat humans and lessen the burden of pain from diseases. There is an art of trusting your doctor and making intelligent choices for yourself to begin healing.

First, focus on getting physical recovery, then follow by seeking emotional support and spiritual help. We may never know why we suffer with physical pain. It is not the field of pathology or pathologists' point of view to believe in God. I personally believe in God, who is often silent on why people suffer. But one thing is true — we can become more mature through the pain in life. At some point, death is inevitable, but until then, we should strive to live with hope and love in God. Even in death which we humans identify as a failure or a dread, there may be glory in God's eye.

Ask and keep on asking and it will be given to you; seek and keep on seeking and you will find; knock and keep on knocking and the door will be opened to you.
— Matthew 7:7

Acknowledgements

I am grateful for Dr. Michael Kanter, who provided important perspectives as a medical school leader who is actively engaged with clinical training of our emerging physicians. Your keen insights integrating the social and economic experiences of patients, and suggestions for clinical implications of pathologists, helped me immensely.

My former UCLA colleague and remarkable surgeon, Dr. Helena Chang, contributed wonderful comments. Her care and kindness for patients is boundless.

Claudia G., your experience and input as a cancer survivor is cherished. Your honest and detailed feedback improved the flow and structure of the entire book.

Sydney Crews, as a pre-medical student, you were so generous with your time while at the University of Oregon. Thank you for reading the manuscript and making insightful, detailed notations in nearly every chapter.

Stephanie Robinson, thank you again for volunteering to help my husband with the production artwork on my books.

To my husband Hal, thank you for the expertise and dedication to publish this book. This book would never be read without your assistance.

Special thanks for my patients, who I serve with gratitude. It is my hope that this book may be helpful to you, your family and friends, or others who face the challenges of cancer.

"Information and knowledge empower us the ability to handle the challenges."

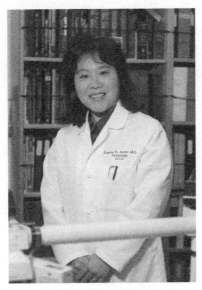

Dr. Apple

Sophia K. Apple, MD, contracted the polio virus as an infant in South Korea and was unable to attend school for nearly four years because of the stigma from her disability. She came to America at age 13 with no knowledge of English, eventually completing medical school. Dr. Apple is a pathologist and expert in breast cancer, Professor Emerita at the David Geffen School of Medicine at UCLA and practices pathology at a large Southern California hospital. She is an author of over 70 peer-reviewed medical journal articles and primary editor of *Breast Imaging*, a medical textbook correlating imagery from pathology and radiology to enhance the quality of breast cancer diagnosis. Dr. Apple is an internationally recognized speaker, and current Editorial Board member of *Modern Pathology*.

Dr. Apple writes novels attributed to "Medicine meeting God," including *COVID-19, a gripping novel inspired by real events,* and *Forgive to Live*. She and her husband currently live in Southern California.

Made in the USA
Monee, IL
12 July 2022

99521841R00059